AIR CRASHES
AND
MIRACLE LANDINGS
PART 1

Large Print Edition

Air Crashes and Miracle Landings is a great resource for every pilot who wants a clear summary of the whats, hows, and whys behind the key aviation accidents. This book should be part of Human Factors and Crew Resource Management training.

Richard de Crespigny
Captain of QF32

AIR CRASHES
AND
MIRACLE LANDINGS
PART 1
Large Print Edition

by

Christopher Bartlett

ISBN 978-0-9560723-7-5
© March 2019

OpenHatch Books,
Gillingham, Dorset, UK
mail@openhatchbooks.com
https://chrisbart.com

Cover
by
Lysa Bartlett

PREFACE

The original Air *Crashes and Miracle Landings*, with all 85 key incidents, remains the ideal Quick Reference Handbook (QRH) for professionals or even fans of the *Air Accident Investigations/MAYDAY* TV series. Having the whole book in one volume facilitates searches, especially on the Kindle.

On the other hand, readers going right through the printed book studying the whys and hows in detail will perhaps prefer this *large-type* edition. A good present for those who remember the headlines at the time and always wondered what really happened.

Chapters 1-7 of the original book are in Part 1, and Chapters 8-18 in Part 2. Updates and the glossary (which we had to omit for lack of space) are in Part 3 for which there is also a Kindle version.

For
all those who died
and
all those who survived.

Lessons
were learned
for the benefit
of us all.

Table of Contents

FIGURES

Diagrams and images are included only where essential for explanation, since so many, even in color or as videos, can be easily found on the Internet.

Chapter 1
LOSS OF POWER
OVER WATER

The Amelia Earhart Mystery (Howland Island, 1937)

America's "favorite missing person"

> Aviatrix Amelia Earhart fully deserved her celebrity status, even though it initially came about fortuitously when in 1928 she was offered the opportunity to be the first woman to fly across the Atlantic after the one initially chosen pulled out fearing the flight was too perilous.
>
> Her life up until then had been no bed of roses. She fell seriously ill during the 1918 Spanish flu pandemic, her family had financial difficulties, and she strove hard in many domains, including aviation where, as always, she tried to further the position of women. On what was to be her last major exploit, an equatorial round the world flight, in 1937, she got two-thirds of the way but then failed to reach a minuscule island in the middle of the Pacific Ocean. Ever since, people have been wondering what happened to her and her navigator.

Earhart later commented she had been little more than a sack of potatoes on that 1928 transatlantic flight. However, the sack must have had grit and courage, as just crossing the Atlantic was a difficult and extremely risky thing to do at the time. Also, the aircraft had to be flown by instruments, something for which she had not at the time been trained, and hence her input limited. Even so, on their return to Manhattan, she and the two male pilots received a ticker-tape welcome, with her seen as a plucky young woman and getting top billing.

Her fame further increased when, in 1932, she became the second person after Charles Lindberg to fly solo across the Atlantic. Though her fifteen-hour flight from Newfoundland to Ireland was much shorter than Lindberg's historic thirty-three-hour flight in 1927 from Long Island to Paris, it proved a considerable ordeal, with icing problems and leaking fuel splashing onto her face.

With the help of her husband, publisher G. P. Putnam, she had stepped on a publicity treadmill, involving a grueling lecture schedule and a constant need to find trailblazing feats to stay in the headlines and keep the money coming in. In the summer of 1937, aged forty and probably somewhat jaded, she was going to embark on what should have been her last major flying exploit, an eastward around-the-world flight along the equator in a Lockheed Electra twin-engine airliner fitted with extra fuel tanks in place of the passenger seats.

She and Putnam were mortgaged to the hilt despite financing from Purdue University. An earlier mishap when taking off in the Electra from Honolulu on their initial attempt to make the around-the-world trip in a westerly direction had added to their costs. On their second attempt, a change in the trade winds forced them to make it in an easterly direction.

Accompanying her on the trip in the key role of navigator was ex–Pan Am navigator Fred Noonan. While reports that he was fired from the airline for a drink problem are disputed, he was an exceptionally capable navigator and an expert at celestial navigation.

Starting from Oakland, California, Earhart and Noonan flew to Miami and then on to Brazil before crossing the narrowest part of the Atlantic to Dakar. After crossing Africa, they flew on to Pakistan, Burma, Singapore, and Darwin in Northern Australia. At times Earhart was quite sick with dysentery, and she must have been exhausted when she arrived at Lae, Papua New Guinea, after the short hop from Darwin. Lae was the departure point for the long transpacific legs, first to tiny Howland Island, and from there on to Hawaii.

Noonan was none too happy, and after an argument with Amelia at Lae apparently went on a drinking spree. When her husband, back in the States, heard about it, he reportedly urged her to call off the venture. She was reluctant to do so, as they had successfully flown twenty-two thousand miles and only had seven thousand to go, and she thought the hardest part had been accomplished.

Whatever his condition, Noonan must have been quite daunted by the prospect of navigating over water with no landmarks to an island only 1.6 square kilometers in area, rising only a foot or two above the sea.

Interestingly, it was the introduction of flying boats in the early thirties that enabled the United States to take over a number of essentially uninhabited islands from the British, which, in the case of Howland, it did only in 1935.

Having jurisdiction at this convenient midway point between Lae and Hawaii in 1937, the US government had prepared a landing strip on the island especially for Amelia's benefit. A US coast guard cutter was also ordered to stand by nearby to render assistance.

Unfortunately, the published coordinates for Howland were out by some five or six miles.

For navigational reasons, Amelia and Noonan timed their departure from Lae so they would fly over land and various identifiable islands in daylight, and then fly overnight over the ocean to Howland, arriving there just after dawn. This meant that while over the ocean and far from land, Noonan would be able to check their position from the stars, provided the weather was not too cloudy. Even after dawn, with no stars to get a fix, Noonan would be able to determine longitude but not latitude by how far the sun was above the horizon for the time of day.

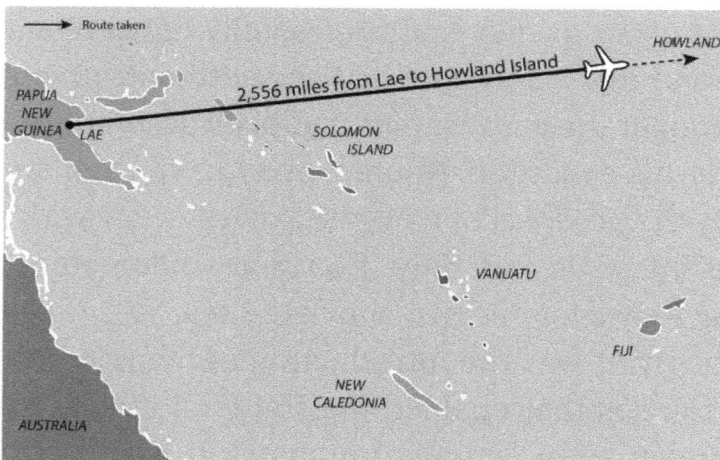

From Lae, Papua New Guinea, to minuscule Howland Island

He would also be using dead reckoning, whereby one's position is calculated according to one's speed, direction of travel, and elapsed time.

As one's actual speed and direction over the ground, as opposed to through the air, depend on the direction and speed of the wind, the method can introduce considerable errors over long distances. Of course, for dead reckoning, correct identification of the waypoints is essential, and as mentioned below it seems Amelia and Noonan misidentified a ship as one that was meant to serve as a waypoint, partly due to their inability to communicate by radio.

The classic way to compensate for the limitations of dead reckoning is to purposely aim for a point well to the left or right of one's destination and, on completing the required distance, make the ninety-degree turn to the right or left to find it. Provided the offset is enough to allow for the navigational error, this avoids the risk of arriving just off to the side of one's destination and flying farther and farther away from it in that direction.

One point that has been rarely made is that Noonan was working under difficult conditions in that the Electra's cabin was crammed with extra fuel tanks, and to get a sighting from the cockpit he would have to clamber, with difficulty, over them. It was also alleged that Earhart's husband, Putnam, had discouraged the idea of Noonan spending time in the cockpit lest it gave the impression that success was down to him.

Getting a sighting from the small window that he had at the back was not easy either and may have contributed to his making errors and their possibly going beyond Howland before turning onto their line of position.

Takeoff from Lae

Laden with maximum fuel for the 2,556-mile leg to Howland, the Electra labored into the air[1] at precisely 00:00 GMT (10:00 a.m. local time) on July 2, 1937. It seems that only the ground effect (air sandwiched between the wings and the ground acting as a cushion[2]) kept them in the air until they were able to raise the wheels to gain enough airspeed to climb away.

When they were four hours eighteen minutes out, Earhart radioed an airport manager back at Lae that they were flying at seven thousand feet and 140 knots, which was ideal for the most efficient consumption of fuel. However, at five hours out she had to climb to avoid a storm and, in the process, used up extra fuel, since, unlike modern airliners, fuel consumption was greater[3] at high altitudes.

Worse was to come. In her hourly call made when seven hours out from Lae, she said that the headwind was 25 knots rather than the 12 knots she had anticipated. If her effective speed was 12 knots slower than her expected ground speed of 140 − 12 = 128 knots, this headwind meant almost a 10 percent increase in the distance through the air.

She seemed to have increased engine power to increase airspeed and optimize her ground distance covered per gallon, but there was certainly still a very significant fuel penalty due to the headwind. Though she was able to call Lae for the first part of the trip, there is no indication she was able to receive any message from Lae in return.

The US government had placed a ship, the *Ontario*,[4] at the halfway point, but it seems that though Earhart and Noonan saw a ship, it was another one forty miles farther north. This may have resulted in them thinking they were on the correct course when in fact they were heading to an area north of Howland Island. (A message she had wanted to send to the *Ontario* before leaving Lae regarding the radio signals the ship should emit had not reached it.)

Howland Island

As the Electra got farther from Lae and nearer Howland, the coast guard cutter *Itasca*, waiting just off the island, began to receive some messages but could not contact them.

Finally, at 7:42 a.m., nineteen and a half hours after their departure from Lae, the *Itasca* received the following message from the Electra:

> *KHAQQ calling Itasca.*
> *We must be on you but cannot see you... Gas is running low... Been unable to reach you by radio. We are flying at one thousand feet.*

Indeed, the signal was so loud the radio operator expected to see them overhead. However, there was no sign of them. The transmission had not lasted long, and the *Itasca* could not get a fix—some say because its direction finder was not working. The *Itasca* emitted smoke, and had there been no cloud, the Electra could have flown higher and seen them from fifty miles.

An hour later, at 8:44 a.m., there was a message in which, according to Doris L. Rich's biography[5], "Amelia's voice—shrill and breathless, her words tumbling over one another—came in."

We are on the line of position 157-337[6]. Will repeat message... We are running north and south.

This final transmission was strong, but not as strong as the earlier one where the operator thought she must be overhead,

The Search

When nothing more was heard, it became increasingly obvious that the Electra must have come down somewhere.

The crew on board the *Itasca* searched the area where they thought they might have been, but there was no sign of them, not even wreckage. The nearest land to Howland Island was 325 miles away, so if Earhart had indeed been as near Howland as she thought she was, there was little chance of her having reached any other land. Some later alleged she had left their life raft behind to save weight.

On President Roosevelt's orders, a major search was launched, involving nine US Navy ships and sixty-six aircraft, at a cost of $4 million or more. They searched a vast area of the Pacific, including the various islands where some people suggested they might have come down. When the authorities finally called off the search after two weeks, the rumors began.

One rumor was that Earhart was a spy for the US government. Hardly anyone believes this to be true now. In the author's view, she would have been much better prepared, especially regarding the use of the radio, had she been a spy. One theory with much traction in the form of witness statements is that she came down on Mili Atoll, to the northwest of Howland, where she and Nolan, suspected as spies, were captured by the Japanese and taken, with their aircraft, to Saipan, where they died. According to witnesses, the embarrassed US government engaged in a major cover-up operation.

During the search, radio messages seeming to emanate from Earhart, some of which caused the US Navy to change the focus of its searches, were received. While many were obviously hoaxes, the navy could not be certain that some were not genuine. Subsequently, a woman's shoe was found on an island she might possibly have reached, only for it to be found not to be her size.

Books and Theories

There are fifty or more books, any number of magazine and newspaper articles and TV documentaries, not to mention online forums, covering her disappearance. The 2009 movie *Amelia* put some meat on the bones of her personal life and her affair with Gene Vidal.

The dashing Gene Vidal was a West Point[7] quarterback who had also come seventh in the 1924 Olympic Games pentathlon and was a prominent figure in aviation. He also happened to be the father of the late Gore Vidal.

In an interview[8] with Robert Chalmers writing for the UK's *The Independent* newspaper, Gore Vidal mentioned that he once asked his father why he had not married Earhart, to which his father replied, "I have never really wanted to marry another boy." Gore Vidal went on to say, "And she was like a boy." He then drew Chalmers's attention to a photo of her in a prominent place on a dresser, remarking, "You see how one could see courage in those eyes," and made it clear how much he admired her and even felt deeply for her.

Searchers have spent tremendous sums trying to locate her aircraft on relatively close islands, such as Nikumaroro, and underwater near Howland. Recently, more credence has been given to some of the radio messages received after her disappearance purporting to be from her. Though searchers are truly fascinated, there is a profit motive. Anyone who succeeds in finding the lost Electra could put the artifacts on show and write the definitive book about her disappearance.

Tom Crouch, senior curator of aeronautics at the National Air and Space Museum, in Washington, who perhaps like others feels he has devoted more than enough time to the case, has said, "I'm convinced that the mystery is part of what keeps us interested. In part, we remember her because she's our favorite missing person." One might push curator Crouch's argument further by saying that people even enjoy arguing about the clues, some of which may have been spun to show the parties, and notably officialdom, in a better light.

Furthermore, some dispute facts once taken as gospel,[9] such as that navigator Noonan was a true alcoholic fired from Pan Am, it being pointed out that he seemed in good form in pictures of him helping Amelia into the aircraft at Lae. Even the idea that the coast guard cutter *Itasca* could have produced a meaningful column of smoke is disputed, since doing so for any significant time would have compromised one of the vessel's boilers, and any smoke would have quickly dissipated in the prevailing wind.

That said, any reader hooked on the subject should note that local time at Howland is GMT plus ten and a half hours, and that this half-hour step can be confusing when comparing times at other places, such as Lae. What is somewhat unsettling is that the great strength of the transmission "We must be on you but cannot see you . . . Gas is running low . . . " gave the impression they were very close.

As mentioned, it even made the *Itasca*'s wireless operator think she might be right overhead and certainly indicated that Noonan had brought her quite close to the minuscule, low-profile Howland Island (whose published coordinates were, as said, out by five or six miles). What's more, her final transmission, at 8:44 a.m., was at maximum strength.

This signal strength, and the later statement "We are running north and south," suggest that she was so determined to reach Howland that she kept trying to get there by going back and forth rather than at some point continuing southward on that line of position, which would very likely have taken them over other islands. Of course, if she waited too long, reaching any other island would be impossible.

Here and elsewhere, commentators have emphasized the general use of the already-mentioned *offset navigation technique*, whereby one aims to one side of one's destination. On reflection, there is a problem with this in the Earhart context. Firstly, when Amelia Earhart says at the outset "We must be on you but cannot see you," it seems to imply they had flown directly to where they thought Howland was. The final message had been

We are on the line of position 157-337. Will repeat message... We are running north and south.

Noonan would have first determined the position of this line when the sun had risen some two hours earlier (see endnote reference to an Internet explanation of the significance of 157-337 degrees) and added to the extra time required so that the line would traverse Howland.

If the unexpected headwinds had not delayed them, the dead reckoning element would have been much reduced.

One interesting theory[10] about what could have gone wrong navigationally is that Noonan got the date wrong for his calculations on approaching Howland Island after crossing the International Date Line. Just before they crossed it at 6 a.m. local time, when he would have been exhausted tired after almost eighteen hours flying, he would have been feverishly trying to get his last star fixes before dawn using the figures in the tables for July 3. Then, just after crossing it he would have been anxious not to miss getting that essential fix on the rising sun.

Could fatigue, stress and fixation on the various tasks have made him forget to switch back to July 2? If so, their position would have been out by one degree of longitude or sixty nautical miles; and with Howland mapped 6 miles out of position, that would have made them think they were at Howland when 66 miles away—too far to see but near enough for the radio signal to have been so strong.

What Earhart perhaps had not realized was that the chances of finding Howland visually in less-than-perfect weather would anyway be slim. In fact, the weather was far from ideal that day, and the only sure way of finding the island would have been by the radio direction finder. In addition, her lack of fuel might have tempted her to try to fly straight to Howland rather than safely to one side to avoid flying away from it.

Everything thus depended on the ability to communicate by radio and the transmission of radio signals on frequencies that respective radio direction finders could pick up. Apparently, there was a lack of coordination between her and the coast guard prior to the flight. The coast guard later tried to portray her as a prima donna unwilling to listen to reason, leading some to interpret this to mean she was a spy unwilling to obey orders from the conventional military.

Though some contemporary female pilots were highly critical of her flying abilities, General Leigh Wade, who had flown with her, claimed she was a born flier "with a delicate touch on the stick." The movie clip—the real one, not the simulated Amelia movie one— showing how she managed the difficult takeoff from Lae, with the aircraft so heavy with extra fuel that it could hardly get off the ground, seems to bear that out. Many a pilot would have pushed the nose up too far and stalled the aircraft. However, there was an early incident in her flying career where her judgment was in question in that she dropped down through cloud not realizing what would have happened had the cloud extended right to the ground.

Anyway, she would have been very reluctant to give up, as she and husband Putnam would be very unlikely to get their money back after a failed exploit. From a modern airline safety point of view, she at first seems to have been silly not to turn back to Lae when she found the climb to a higher altitude and the unexpected increase in headwind meant she would have little fuel in reserve even if she made a perfect course to Howland.

However, going back to Lae would have involved going again over nine-thousand-foot peaks on Bougainville Island, in the Solomon Islands.

What is more, the takeoff from Lae, even though helped by the headwind that later caused her to use more fuel than expected, had been a touch-and-go affair, and she might not have been so lucky a second time. Lack of high-octane aviation fuel on the island would mean waiting until further supplies arrived and paying for their shipment.

Weather conditions might be even worse the next time, and there was no guarantee the US Navy would keep the Itasca on station at Howland. Finally, she could not be sure the Electra could withstand another takeoff at one and half times its normal maximum takeoff weight.

On her other flights toward large landmasses, having ample reserves of fuel was not so critical—for instance, on her transatlantic solo flight she was said to have been hoping to emulate Charles Lindbergh's 1927 historic flight from New York's Long Island to Le Bourget Field, Paris, and yet ended up in Ireland, both large landmasses.

Her, some might say, forgotten navigator, the recently married Noonan, must also have had considerable courage to embark on the venture. Were the fatigue and stress getting to her and making her disapprove of his conduct, or was he unhappy about preparations for the particularly difficult flight ahead?

View a Modern Air Accident Inquiry Would Take

A modern air accident inquiry might say the direct causes of the tragedy, apart from the inherent risk, included:

1. Failure to master the use of radio communication and particularly radio direction-finding technology (RDF), failure to ensure it was set up and tested properly, and failure to check the compatibility of the radio and direction-finding equipment.

2. Failure to employ backup Morse code radio equipment (with its direction-finding features), perhaps on account of failure to master Morse code.

Allegedly she had dispensed with a loop antenna to save weight. Others say it struck something and fell off on taking off from Lae. The fact that a couple of people who were to participate in the earlier aborted attempt in an easterly direction were no longer available, plus a lack of funds, probably meant the venture was not professionally managed, resulting in a lack of liaison between the parties, especially regarding use of the radio equipment.

Even had the *Itasca* been able to get an RDF fix, it would not have enabled it to give her the vector to reach Howland, as she was not receiving its transmissions. It would, though, have given some general idea of where to look for her—then and even now.

The Search Goes On

For eighty years people in the United States and all over the world have been speculating on what happened to Amelia and Noonan, but nowadays the main impetus for endeavors to find her aircraft comes from an organization called TIGHAR (pronounced "tiger"), standing for The International Group for Historic Aircraft Recovery. Its members donate funds for searches, with them now focusing on Nikumaroro Atoll (also called Gardner Island) on the line of position 157-337, passing through Howland but two hours' flying time to the south.

They are not the first to look for Amelia-related items there, and previous seekers have found artifacts made from aluminum, some from a B-24.

In 1940, a partial skeleton was discovered but dismissed when a British doctor said it was of a male. The island was then part of the British Gilbert and Ellice Islands Crown Colony.

The bones disappeared, but the doctor had taken notes, and TIGHAR recently got two forensic anthropologists— Karen Burns, PhD, and Richard Jantz, PhD—to review them. They concluded that "the morphology of the recovered bones, insofar as we can tell by applying contemporary forensic methods to measurements taken at the time, appears consistent with a female of Earhart's height and ethnic origin."

However, other experts are inclined to agree with finding made by the British doctor in 1940 that the bones were those of a male.

TIGHAR also are giving increased credence to radio transmissions, purportedly from Amelia after she had come down, that were picked up by a sixteen-year-old girl radio ham in Texas and a woman in Melbourne, listening on a harmonic of the frequency Amelia used.

One has to wonder why Earhart and Noonan with hardly any remaining fuel would go down as far as Nikumaroro Atoll, almost 400 miles (640 kilometers) away from Howland.

For TIGHAR to keep the pot boiling and funds coming in for further missions with a submersible to explore around Nikumaroro, it is only natural for them to constantly come up with—as they always do—new reasons to hope Amelia's aircraft wreckage will soon be found. Its pronouncements are picked up by the world's media and published almost verbatim for a fascinated public. However doubtful one may be, one still gets hooked.

For one highly dubious skeptic's correspondence with TIGHAR's Gillespie see:
https://earharttruth.wordpress.com/tag/nikumaroro/
In 2017, the National Geographic Channel had a program about Amelia Earhart showing a photo purportedly of her and Nolan on a pier, implying she had been captured by the Japanese. However, a researcher in

Japan found the photo in question in a book published two years before her disappearance!

Until hard evidence or the wreck of her Electra is found, people will always wonder.

As curator Tom Crouch said, "She is our favorite missing person."

──────────────────

[1] http://www.tighar.org/amelia_3.rm is a 30-second clip of the takeoff. It shows Earhart and Noonan apparently looking fit when boarding. Also, see www.tighar.org.

[2] To describe the ground effect as simply a cushioning effect is an oversimplification, as the aerodynamics are much more complicated.

[3] Amelia Earhart: The Mystery Solved, Elgen M. Long, Marie K. Long.

[4] http://www.thehistorynet.com/ahi/blearhart/index3.html.

[5] Amelia Earhart: A Biography, by Doris L. Rich.

[6] Best explanation of significance of "157-337." http://tighar.org/forum/FAQs/navigation.html

[7] US military academy

[8] Interview by Robert Chalmers, *The Independent*, 25 May, 2008.

[9] See http://www.tighar.org/forum/FAQs/Forumfaq.html

[10] See datelinetheory.com

Captain Coolly Announces No Engines Working (Jakarta, 1982)
Out-of-this-world phenomenon

> In 1982, a British Airways 747 encountered a strange, almost mystical phenomenon high up in the lonely sky off Indonesia. With the aircrew not knowing why, all four engines failed, leaving the aircraft gliding through the night sky, with high mountains between them and the nearest diversion airport, and the Indian Ocean below.
>
> British Airways Flight 9, June 24, 1982

M any of the passengers—and particularly those who had boarded in London and endured multiple stops and delays on what was then the longest scheduled five-stopover flight, from London to New Zealand—were dozing off after the evening meal. Everything had been going smoothly on that leg from Kuala Lumpur to Perth, Australia, with only one more stopover to go.

Then some two and a half hours into the leg, passengers on the Boeing 747 started complaining that there were too many smokers. On seeing the haze at the back of the economy-class cabin, the cabin crew wondered why so many were lighting up when they would normally be trying to get some sleep. As the smoke and acrid smell of burning increased, cabin staff surreptitiously went around ensuring a smoldering cigarette was not about to start a fire.

Meanwhile, profiting from a quiet moment on the flight deck, the captain had taken the opportunity to go to the toilet and stretch his legs. The first officer and flight engineer left in charge on the flight deck had the autopilot handling the aircraft and only needed to keep a lookout and be ready for anything unexpected.

Having passed right over Indonesia's capital, Jakarta, the 747 was about to cross the mountains and head out over the Indian Ocean, stretching from India to Antarctica. Cruising at thirty-seven thousand feet, with bright stars overhead and little cloud below, the first officer and flight engineer began to see odd light effects ahead, which they later said were like Saint Elmo's fire, a phenomenon in which lightning dances around in the sky. Yet their weather radar gave no indication of storm clouds.

Soon, with flashes of light and tiny balls of fire rushing at them and exploding on the windscreen, the crew's amazement switched to concern, and the first officer called the captain, who was relaxing just below. Hurrying up the stairs, Captain Moody could hardly believe what he was seeing. No one could work out what it was; it seemed out of this world. High up in the sky, with no light pollution, anything producing some degree of light is immediately obvious, and a strange glow seemed to be enveloping the leading edge of the wings and the nacelles of the engines. Worse still, the engines themselves appeared to be illuminated from inside. Passengers seated behind the engines were startled to see bright particles issuing from them. Their rough running began to rouse the few passengers still asleep.

A pungent smell of smoke prompted the flight engineer to check for fire and consider shutting down the air-conditioning, even though he could not find any reason to do so.

Two minutes after entering the zone where the strange phenomenon was occurring, the instruments indicated a pneumatic valve pressure problem for the number four (outside right) engine, which afterward surged and flamed out. A minute later the number two engine failed likewise, and failure of engines number one and three soon followed. They had become a glider with 15 crew members and 248 passengers, including children and babies.

Though airliners do not make good gliders, their great cruising height—in this case thirty-seven thousand feet—means they usually have some time in which to restart the engines or select somewhere they might be able to land in the most unlikely event of the engines failing at cruising height. However, in this case their predicament was particularly serious in that the nearest diversion airport (Jakarta-Halim) had high mountains on its approach, and it would be quite impossible to keep above the 11,500-foot minimum height needed to reach it safely.

Ditching a 747 in the sea in daytime when able to judge the height and direction of the swell would be difficult enough, but it was 10 p.m., and the chances of a successful ditching in the dark would be virtually zero, especially as unknown to them at the time their landing lights had been sandblasted and would have been useless. While any survivors might find the warm waters of the Indian Ocean more hospitable than, say, the cold Atlantic, the likelihood of someone bleeding would mean it would not be long before sharks came for a late supper.

The flight engineer made repeated attempts to restart the engines, much to the consternation of the passengers at the rear of the aircraft, who saw burning fuel mixed with whatever had accumulated in the engines spewing out explosively each time.

With no power for cabin pressurization, the air pressure inside the aircraft was gradually dropping. After about five minutes it fell so much that the crew had to don their oxygen masks, not only because of their physical exertion but because they needed all their mental faculties, and the human brain uses a surprising amount of oxygen. It was only then that the first officer found his oxygen mask had been stowed incorrectly and was unusable, forcing them to drop down from 26,000 feet to 20,000 feet for his benefit.

As they lost further valuable height and sank to 17,500 feet, with the cabin pressure still falling, the passengers' oxygen masks descended.

The situation seemed to be becoming more and more critical. Little did they know their imposed loss of height would be their salvation. Almost twelve minutes after losing all power, they found themselves nosing into normal air below the unnatural zone.

Shortly afterward, the first engine they had shut down, and the least subjected to whatever the cause was, sprang into life.

One engine alone would not provide enough power for them to climb but would keep them aloft for much longer and give them some measure of control over their destiny. Subsequently, the other three engines also came back to life in quick succession.

Rather prematurely they reported this reprieve to the tower controller at Jakarta, who told them to climb to fifteen thousand feet, as the mountains between them and the airport were making them invisible to the Jakarta radar. In complying, they found themselves yet again in the abnormal zone, and one of the resurrected engines begun to run so roughly that they had to shut it down. They lost no time in dropping down into the clear air again.

With careful nursing, the three other engines seemed to be sustaining their power. Thinking their tribulations were over, they approached the airport at Jakarta in high spirits, only to find the "sandblasted" windscreen had frosted over so much that everything was a blur.

They even had to request that the tower decrease the intensity of the runway lights because of the glare. Fortunately, each windscreen panel had a narrow strip of clear glass down each outboard side, allowing them to see just enough to land safely. The captain performed well, making a very good landing with help from the first officer reading out the heights.

One passenger was violently sick due to mental stress as they came in, but all things considered it was surprising more passengers were not similarly indisposed.

The 747's landing at Jakarta had in the end been normal, but in view of the doubtful state of the engines,

Moody asked that they be towed to the terminal, with the passengers thanking God and above all the crew, personified by the captain, for their deliverance.

The odds against all four engines of an aircraft failing for reasons other than fuel depletion are so great that it is—or was—thought to be virtually impossible. However, the aircrew had trained for such an eventuality and performed very competently, as did the cabin crew. The constantly repeated efforts to restart the engines, probably stopped them clogging up completely.

They later learned that what they had encountered had been ash from a volcano, which explained why being forced to lose height due to the first officer's faulty oxygen mask had been such a blessing. Had they spent longer in the ash-laden environment it is conceivable that the engines would have silted up too much to be relit.

Interestingly, it is thought that when the ash fused by the heat of the engine fully cooled it became brittle, then broke off and was ejected. Some would argue the aircrew should have put on their oxygen masks earlier and thereby solved the problem, with the first officer's mask before being obliged to descend. However, not doing so happened to work in their favor.

The authorities closed the skies around the volcano (Mount Galunggung) to aircraft for a week.

Just four days after they were reopened, a Singapore Airlines 747 encountered conditions like those that had caught the BA crew by surprise. Forewarned, the SIA crew took evasive action, but even so had to divert to Jakarta-Halim, as three of their engines had overheated.

There was an almost identical incident in 1989, when a KLM flight from Amsterdam to Anchorage, Alaska, encountered an ash cloud from Mount Redoubt and all four engines flamed out. As in the BA case, the pilots were able to restart them on exiting the plume of ash.

In a commendation ceremony for both the aircrew and cabin crew, BA was happy to bathe in the reflected glory. Captain Eric Moody, later left the airline to become a TV pundit on aviation matters and a much-in-demand after-dinner speaker.

In a deftly written review of the TV documentary *All Engines Failed*, the UK's *Daily Mail* said Moody "displayed the stiff-upper-lip spirit that built an empire" when he uttered the words that are every air passenger's worst nightmare: "Ladies and gentlemen, this is your captain speaking. We have a small problem. All four engines have stopped. We are doing our damnedest to get it under control. I trust you are not in too much distress."

The crisis resolved itself thanks to difficulties with the first officer's oxygen mask forcing Moody to bring the aircraft down to uncontaminated air where the engines could restart before silting up completely. When all engines flame out (stop), pilots are loath to gratuitously cede height, as that lessens the time available to restart them.

To be fair, the captain's calm demeanor and theatrically delivered words not only reassured the passengers but must have helped the crew perform optimally in the testing circumstances.

The strain Moody was under in the sky above the Indian Ocean and the ramifications career-wise are perhaps evident from the fact that a year later his hair had turned completely white. How pilots cope with the instant notoriety and PTSD arising from such events is often overlooked amidst the adulation and awe. Relations with colleagues can become strained.

Nowadays, more help is at hand. For example, Sullenberger who famously ditched his Airbus A320 in the Hudson River tells how he could not sleep or think normally for quite some time afterward but got advice about what would happen mentally that proved correct. He said talking about the incident was a great help— something that might well apply to Richard de Crespigny who wrote a book about QF32 (see Chapter 10 in Part 2) and gives lectures and talks.

Pilot Struggling with Hijacker Ditches off Beach (Comoros, 1996)

Within sight of bathers; video seen around the world

> The Ethiopian pilot was fighting off a hijacker, had insufficient electrical power and thus only limited control of the aircraft.
>
> Ethiopian Airlines Flight 961, November 23, 1996

In 1996, an Ethiopian Airlines Boeing 767 was seized by three hijackers, who thought that the range quoted in the in-flight magazine meant it could fly all the way to Australia, when in fact the pilots had only loaded enough fuel for the leg in question, which was a quarter of the distance.

Even though the pilots explained this was not possible they thought they were being tricked and insisted on going on. In an impossible situation, the captain, Leul Abate, tried to keep within sight of the African coast, but the hijackers noticed this. Pretending he was complying and going out toward the open sea, the captain flew toward the Comoros Islands. Fuel was running out when they neared them, but this did not prevent the hijackers remonstrating with the pilots and preventing them from landing at the main airport.

Struggling with the hijackers, Abate lost track of the way to the airport and with one engine having flamed out due to fuel depletion, opted to ditch in the sea just off a beach with possible help at hand. The second engine then flamed out, and with no electrical power to set the flaps, he was anyway coming in too fast. He wanted to come down parallel to the waves, but at the last moment a hijacker grabbed the controls, causing the left wingtip to dip and snag the water and the aircraft to spin leftward. The left engine hit the water and then allegedly a reef, causing the aircraft to cartwheel and break up.

Of the 175 crew and passengers, only 48, including Captain Abate but not the hijackers, survived.

Premature inflation of life jackets, despite a warning not to do so, was the cause of many fatalities. Besides their bulk making it more difficult for people to get out, prematurely inflated life jackets can cause the wearer to float upwards if the cabin fills with water, resulting in their being trapped.

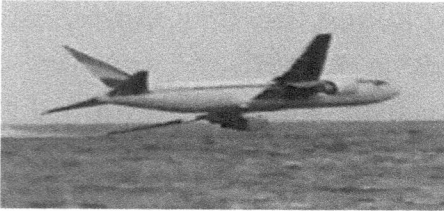

Wingtip touches the water, then the engine

Though the hijackers claimed to be eight in number, there were only three, and their bombs were fake.

Leul Abate had already experienced two hijackings, which had ended with no loss of life. He claimed his copilot was the real hero, for even though injured he continued to wrestle with the by-then-suicidal hijackers, giving him some respite to maneuver the aircraft.

A330 Glides Eighty Miles Over Atlantic to an Island (Azores, 2001)
The longest airliner glide ever

> Switching to today's ETOPS era, with some twin-engine aircraft allowed to fly as much as three hours flying time from a suitable landing place, we have an instance where an airliner ran out of fuel over the Atlantic.
>
> They were eighty miles from the nearest landing place, a US military airfield on an island in the Azores. Reaching it was one thing; adjusting height and speed so as not to overshoot or undershoot and come down in the sea was quite another.
>
> Air Transat Flight 236, August 24, 2001

The Air Transat Airbus A330 en route over the Atlantic from Toronto to Lisbon was only two years old but had had the right engine changed five days before. Cruising at 39,000 feet, with 293 passengers and 13 crew, air traffic control had instructed them to fly a route 60 kilometers further south than usual to avoid congestion.

The captain who had had a colorful past was 48-year-old Robert Piché with 16,800 flight hours, and the copilot 28-year-old First Officer Dirk DeJager with 4,800 flight hours.

Some four hours into the flight the computer (ECAM) warned about a low oil temperature and high oil pressure for the right engine. Since it was so unusual the pilots sought the advice of their company's maintenance department back in Canada, but they too were puzzled and could not offer any help. This opened the possibility in the pilots' minds that the instruments might be playing up.

Twenty minutes later the ECAM warned of a developing imbalance between the amount of fuel in the inner fuel tanks in the left and right wing, with less in the right wing. The pilots activated the cross-feed to transfer fuel from the left tank to the one in the right wing, only to find it was not correcting the imbalance.

On calculating their fuel consumption, First Officer DeJager found they had used more than they should have. Knowing it could be due to a fuel leak Captain Piché ordered a flight attendant to check the wings from the passenger cabin window and was informed there is no sign of one—it was dark, and the fuel would have been coming out low down.

If the instrument readings were correct, they would not have enough fuel to reach Lisbon, their destination, and would have to divert. Air traffic informed them that the nearest suitable runway was at a US air base called Lajes in the Azores 300 kilometers away, which they had ample fuel to reach.

Piché altered course and headed for Lajes, all the while wondering whether diverting was necessary, and it was not merely partly a matter of faulty instruments. Then, just over half an hour from the time they had the first fuel imbalance warning the right engine flamed out due to lack of fuel.

The pilots applied full power on the left engine but even so had to descend to 33,000 feet as the aircraft could not fly at 39,000 feet on only one engine.

They declared a MAYDAY, even though sure they had ample fuel to reach Lajes, and still wondering whether the computer was partly at fault.

Thirteen minutes after the right engine had flamed out, the left one did likewise, leaving them engineless and with only minimal electrical power supplied by the RAT (Ram Air Turbine), a kind of windmill generator that deploys when the engines cannot generate any electricity.

Carefully nursing his Airbus A330, captain Piché managed to glide to the island and come in at four hundred miles per hour rather than risk falling out of the sky by attempting an extra circuit to lose more height and speed. With no air brakes or flaps, and with only the landing gear to slow him, he raised the nose to decrease the sink rate and increase forward resistance.

Hitting hard near the runway threshold, he burst eight tires. Not because as may assumed because he hit so hard, but because the antilocking system was not functioning and with the wheels locked by the brakes, the tires just skidded over the runway without rotating.

The aircraft with its terrified passengers shuddered to a halt almost three-quarters of the way down the runway. Waiting fire service appliances quickly ensured the sparks resulting from friction between exposed metal wheel rims and the runway did not start a fire, which was unlikely in view of the empty, unruptured fuel tanks and their being empty, though there would have been hydraulic fluid.

All on board evacuated in less than ninety seconds thanks to the excellent work of the cabin crew, whom some passengers later accused of panicking, as they were shouting so loudly—the airline retorted that the crew had to shout to ensure everyone heard them. In fact, some passengers, froze while others tried to bring their hand luggage.

Only twelve passengers sustained injuries in the course of the evacuation, and those were minor. Some were vomiting beside the runway after the tension of the long glide.

On Piché's return to Canada, people showered praise on him, but to one journalist he obliquely replied, "I don't consider myself a hero, sir. I could have done without this." This probably rightly conveyed his sentiment of just having done his job and having been lucky but could also have intimated his fear that details of his prison sentence in the United States for allegedly smuggling marijuana in a light plane in his younger days would leak out.

Before readers jump to conclusions regarding his suitability to be a captain, they should note that in applying for a job with the airline he did not hide that fact. Indeed, in an interview quite some time after his great feat, he claimed the experience of facing death several times as the only French-speaking inmate in an American jail was what had given him the fortitude to make the successful landing after enduring the stress of the long glide.

Investigations subsequently showed the cause of the incident was faulty maintenance by the airline. However, there remained the question as to whether Piché and his first officer aggravated the situation by poor judgment. Were they largely responsible for their own misfortune? Alternatively, had the sophisticated computer systems and displays on the aircraft been at fault?

The Canadian authorities' imposition of a $250,000 fine on Air Transat and the reduction of their ETOPS rating to a maximum diversion time of only ninety minutes attest to the seriousness of the maintenance lapses.

They discovered that on finding metal filings in the oil, engineers temporarily installed the only replacement Rolls-Royce engine they had available on site for loan in such situations—one that happened to be a slightly older version, and one not equipped with a fuel pump. With no pump, they decided to use the existing one fitted to their own newer engine that they were removing, despite the concern expressed by one member of the team.

The airliner had crossed the Atlantic thirteen times since the change to the older model engine without anyone realizing that using parts designed for the newer engine on the older version would allow the fuel line to chafe. On that fourteenth crossing the fuel line ruptured and broke. The fuel kept pouring out of the wing, and even though Captain Piché asked a crew member to check, they were unable to see it in the darkness.

The inquiry's findings were as follows:

1. The main cause was irresponsible maintenance;
2. Piché and his first officer had possibly aggravated the fuel leak situation by making wrong decisions regarding the transfer of fuel between tanks.

Having reviewed the aircraft's computer systems and displays, Airbus took measures to make pilots aware of abnormal fuel consumption even without doing the calculations themselves. They revised the manual to stress the need even further to avoid transferring fuel where any suspicion of a fuel leak existed. Rolls-Royce was the subject of some criticism for putting Air Transat in a difficult situation by not providing the pump together with the engine.

The Pilots' Performance

Being able to glide so far was due not only due to good calculation of the optimum glide slope and avoiding overcontrolling, but also to the aerodynamics of the A330 and the great height at which they were initially flying. Perhaps the key to this success was the way Piché eased the aircraft along and risked coming in too fast rather than losing more height by circling, as it was suggested the first officer wanted to do, and the possibility of having to ditch.

Some commentators have remarked that the aircraft would have toppled over the cliff at the far end of the runway and into the sea had Piché not landed so adroitly. In fact, the "cliff" is an optical illusion when looking along the runway toward the end, as the ground merely slopes downward beyond the runway, giving the impression that it is a sheer drop to the sea. Even had the aircraft been about to go over the so-called cliff, all would not have been lost, as Lajes is a military field, with arresting chains at either end of the runway. Controllers can raise these if an aircraft (with possibly a weapons payload) looks as though it will overrun.

Had there been enough electrical power to keep the flight recorders functioning, investigators would have been able to learn more about the glide and final control inputs. With the batteries drained in the course of the long glide, the ram air turbine (RAT) was providing essential power for the most basic instruments and controls. However, electricity for the flight recorders was not considered essential at the time, though the NTSB now says it should be maintained in all circumstances.

Piché, with his charming, unconventional personality, became a hero, especially in Canada, with hundreds of people wanting to interview him. He was asked to open various events, almost like royalty. He had a biography written about him and spent some time on sick leave, apparently with alcohol problems brought about by the unwanted roller-coaster ride of fame and shame. He then gave up drinking entirely and returned to work as a pilot at the airline.

It is a very human story, made more dramatic by the perception that the landing was on a remote island, which consequently must have poor facilities. As mentioned above, this was not the case. Piché was the first to admit that luck played a part. The weather was almost perfect, unlike the day before and the day after. Air traffic control (ATC) had by chance allotted him a route sixty miles farther south than usual, thus putting him just within gliding range of the Azores when the fuel ran out.

Other pilots have successfully made dead-stick landings, and most of them, including Piché, deserve praise. The question is, to what extent was Piché responsible for his own misfortune?

Culture of the Airline

The culture of the small airline surely played a part. When the fuel imbalance became serious enough to be worrying, it seems the pilots hesitated to divert immediately, as they were wondering what the airline would say if they landed in the Azores with full tanks. Pilots working for a major carrier might not be under such pressure, as their diversion, if finally proven unnecessary, would only be a mere blip compared with the airline's vast scenario of operations.

For a relatively small operation such as Air Transat, the cost of the diversion and schedule disruption would of course have been of concern. Of even greater concern might have been the fear of losing its ETOPS classification through too many diversions for mechanical reasons. As already mentioned, a regulation designed to ensure safety sometimes has the opposite result.

Was There Really a Miracle on the Hudson? (NYC, 2009)

"Everyone is looking for a hero," said Sully on talk show

> In awe of the fairy-tale outcome, we almost all saw this in terms of the captain's heroic achievement: ditching his Airbus A320 in New York City's Hudson River *with not a single life lost.*
>
> Looking more closely, one can see that the "miracle" was not simply the ditching itself—it was more complicated than that.
>
> US Airways Flight 1549, January 15, 2009

Cactus is the call sign air traffic controllers use for US Airways. This seems bizarre until one realizes that was the call sign used by American West Airlines (AWE), with which US Airways merged and which indeed flies to many locations where cacti grow. For air traffic control, the merged airline also kept the American West identification code, AWE.

For the public, the name US Airways was retained, allegedly because it sounded more prestigious, and doing so had the advantage of keeping both parties to the merger happy. Also, there was a lot of confusion both with ATC and passengers over differentiating American and American West. For ATC, it was much better and safer to use Cactus. USAir was always an awkward mouthful anyway for controllers.

After lifting off from LaGuardia's Runway 4 at 3:25:33 p.m. on January 15, 2009, and bound for Charlotte, two hours' flying time away, Cactus 1549 (US Airways 1549) was handed over to departure (control) with clearance to climb to five thousand feet.

Including the two pilots, Captain Chesley Sullenberger ("Sully") and First Officer Jeffrey Skiles, and three cabin crew, there were a hundred and fifty-five people on board the Airbus 320. It was a beautiful day but rather cold.

The only thing unusual about the aircraft was that although it was a domestic inland flight it was equipped with life rafts.

Exchanges with Air Traffic Control (ATC)

To simplify the transcriptions of exchanges between the aircraft and ATC, we refer to US Airways flights as "Cactus" rather than "AWE," and use "Departure" when the full name is "New York TRACOM LaGuardia Departure[1]."

"Departure" was the controller handling flights from climb-out (that is after they had taken off) to the time they reached approximately eighteen thousand feet and were then handed over to the ATC center (in this case New York Center) covering the upper skies for the whole area.

After two or three routine exchanges between Departure and Cactus 1549, Departure gave instructions to turn left as a first step on the two-hour flight to Charlotte.

3:27:32 p.m. Departure:

> *Cactus 1549 turn left heading two seven zero* [i.e. due West]

There was no immediate confirmation from the aircraft, but four seconds later, with a slight error in the call sign indicative of the stressful situation:

3:27:36 p.m. Cactus 1549:

Ah, this is Cactus 1539 [sic] . . . Hit birds. We lost thrust in both engines. We're turning back toward LaGuardia.

Departure:

Okay. Yeah. You need to return to LaGuardia. . . Turn left, heading of, uh, two two zero.

Cactus 1549:

Two two zero.

Departure called the LaGuardia tower, telling them to stop all departures, that the aircraft in trouble was in fact Cactus 1549, and that they had lost all engines. The tower (the local controller) found this difficult to grasp, perhaps because the simultaneous loss of all engines is almost unheard of.

Departure clarified:

Cactus 1549 has lost thrust in both engines.

Tower:

Got it.

Departure to Cactus 1549:

Cactus 1549, if we can get it to you, do you want to try to land Runway 13?

Runway 13 was perpendicular to the one from which Sully had just taken off and had the advantage that aligning with it would be quicker and involve less turning. In a turn an aircraft loses lift and the sink rate increases, and normally extra power has to be applied to compensate.

Cactus 1549:

We're unable. We may end up in the Hudson.

Departure:

All right, Cactus 1549, it's going to be left traffic to Runway 31.

Cactus 1549:

Unable.

Departure:

Okay, what do you need to land?

Departure:

Cactus 1549, Runway 4 is available if you want to make left traffic to Runway 4.

Cactus 1549:

I am not sure if we can make any runway. Oh, what's over to our right? Anything in New Jersey, maybe Teterboro?

(Departure called Teterboro airport on the other side of the Hudson River and told them that LaGuardia Departure had an "emergency inbound" and asked if their Runway 1 would be okay. Approval was given.)

Departure to Cactus 1549:

Cactus 1529 turn right two eight zero. You can land Runway 1 at Teterboro.

Cactus 1549:

We can't do it.

Departure:

Okay. Which runway would you like at Teterboro?

3:29:28 p.m. Last transmission from Cactus 1549:

We're going in the Hudson.

Departure:

I'm sorry, say again, Cactus.

Departure quickly dealt with another aircraft before saying:

Cactus, ah, Cactus 1549, radar contact is lost. You also got Newark airport off your two o'clock and about seven miles.

Having overheard the earlier exchange, the pilot of Eagle 4718 called Departure:

Eagle 4718, I don't know, I think he said he was going in the Hudson.

Though the Manhattan skyscrapers had blocked the echo from the aircraft making it invisible on the Departure controller's radar, it fleetingly reappeared making him wonder whether an engine had revived. On the outside chance that it might be useful, he transmitted information about the runway available at Newark, seven miles ahead of Cactus 1549's presumed position.

Events in the Air

Just before Sullenberger (nickname Sully) reported the bird strike and announced his intention to return to LaGuardia, the Airbus had been climbing through 3,200 feet under takeoff power, with everything quite normal.

The flock of birds appeared from almost nowhere. The first officer, flying the aircraft at the time, saw them first. Sully saw them just as they were about to hit and later said he wanted to duck. They struck the windscreen and other parts of the aircraft with unusually loud thuds, as they were so large. A passenger in first class later said he saw a "gray shape" shoot past his window and go into the engine and that he knew it had done so because of the colossal *bam*. The engines powered down, with another passenger later saying the engines "sounded like a spin dryer with a tennis shoe rolling around in it," according to *The Miracle of the Hudson Plane Crash*, Channel 4 (UK), February 19, 2009.

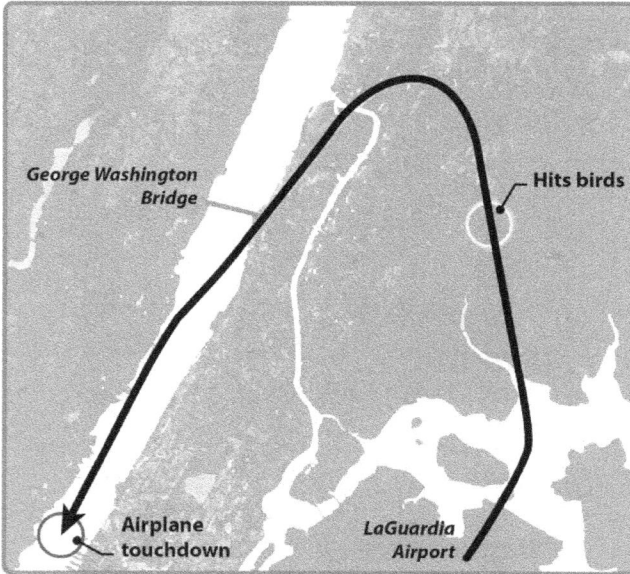

Route followed by the A320 (based on image courtesy of NTSB)

Sully took over control from his first officer, Jeffrey Skiles, with the words "My aircraft," and he or the A320's computer, or both, pushed the nose down so the aircraft would not stall. Interviewed later, on *60 Minutes*, Sully said, "It was the worst, sickening, pit-of-the-stomach, falling-through-the-floor feeling I've ever felt in my life. The physiological reaction I had of this was strong, and I had to force myself to use my training and to force calm on the situation."

As detailed in the transcription above, Sully informed air traffic control (ATC) of the situation and indicated his intention to turn back to LaGuardia, but after dismissing the options of returning to LaGuardia or trying Teterboro, he said he would have to come down in the Hudson. He therefore continued his turn to the left until he was flying along the left bank of the wide river.

He skirted the George Washington Bridge, with its 604-foot (184-meter) twin towers. Manhattan's Central Park was ahead on the left. With the first officer, Skiles, vainly trying to restart an engine using a checklist conceived for dual engine failure at a very much greater height, Sully brought the aircraft over the river itself. He made a single announcement for the benefit of the cabin crew, as well as the passengers:

This is the captain; brace for impact!

The aircraft was at five hundred feet and the time between the captain's announcement and the actual "impact" seemed inordinately long perhaps because the great height of the buildings in Manhattan gave the passengers the impression that they were lower than they really were.

In addition, the A320 was leveling out and losing speed, so it was not traveling so fast on nearing the water.

The flight attendants were following their training, shouting "Brace! Brace! Heads down! Stay down!" in unison at intervals.

One flight attendant later mentioned her concern that some passengers were raising their heads to look out of the windows. This was understandable, as some ninety seconds elapsed between the captain saying, "Brace for impact" and the actual impact. Not realizing "impact" meant one with water, many passengers feared they might do a 9/11—that is, fly straight into a building and end up inside a ball of fire.

Lest we forget the short time frame, Sully only had about three minutes from the time the engines failed to the moment the aircraft would inevitably come down, either under control with the possibility of survival if a suitable spot could be found, or out of control following a stall with very little hope of but a few surviving.

Also, while Sully was concentrating on flying the aircraft, First Officer Jeffrey Skiles wasted valuable time on hopeless attempts to extract some meaningful thrust from the engines, which were still running, but at very low power and were useless. The NTSB investigators later recommended engine makers try to develop some system whereby pilots could assess the nature and extent of damage via their instruments.

The Impact

Sully had successfully restarted the auxiliary power unit (APU) to generate electricity; in addition, the ram air turbine (RAT) had apparently deployed automatically. This meant he had more than adequate power to run his cockpit displays and control systems. For the Airbus A320, the manufacturer recommends Flaps 3 and a minimum approach airspeed of 150 knots, with eleven degrees of pitch at touchdown. According to FDR data, the airplane touched down on the Hudson River at a calibrated airspeed of 125 knots with a pitch angle of 9.5 degrees and a right roll angle of 0.4 degrees.

Calculations indicated that the airplane ditched with a descent rate of 12.5 feet per second, a flightpath angle of –3.4 degrees, an angle of attack between 13 and 14 degrees, and a side slip angle of 2.2 degrees. The lack of airspeed meant Sully could not break the too-rapid sink rate with his flare.

What is certain is that the bottom of the fuselage at the rear struck the water first and sufficiently hard to damage some panels. In consequence, the experiences of those on board differed considerably, with the female flight attendant at the rear possibly getting the worst of it, and the pilots at the front getting the best. Apparently, the two pilots were surprised at how smooth their touchdown had been.

On coming to a halt, the aircraft slewed around, no doubt because only one engine had sheared off. (Aircraft engines slung under the wings are attached in such a way that they will break off under an extreme rearward force, such as in the case of hitting an object when crash-landing, or the water when ditching. This prevents the wing(s) being ripped off.)

Events on the Water

Thankful for how well it had appeared to have gone, at least to the two pilots at the front, they knew that only half the battle had been won. Everything depended now not only on getting everyone out safely but also on their being picked up before the icy water (36°F, or 2°C) of the Hudson River took its toll. Pictures of the passengers standing on the wings so happy to be still alive give the impression the evacuation was something of a picnic. This is far from the truth, particularly for the passengers and the flight attendant at the very rear of the aircraft.

As mentioned, the impact with the water damaged fuselage panels at the rear. Water seeped mainly in from there and not, as some accounts state, from a rear door that had somehow cracked open. A female flight attendant tried to shut it without success. Fit people at the back clambered over seatbacks to escape the influx of water, not knowing whether the situation might suddenly worsen. As they moved forward toward relative safety, the flight attendant who had been at the rear realized for the first time that she might survive.

The first officer had been using a ditching checklist written on the assumption that the decision to ditch would be made at a great height, with plenty of time to prepare. This meant that he did not get as far as the line at the end where it said, "Press the ditching button" (at two thousand feet), which would have closed various vents and the like. Thus, more water than otherwise would have been the case was coming in. Even so, this did not mean the aircraft would immediately sink completely.

Sully had brought the aircraft down between two ferry terminals, and help was soon on its way. Before leaving the aircraft, he walked up and down the aisle twice to make sure no one remained. He then stepped out and told rescuers to save people on the wings first, as he knew the life rafts could stay afloat almost indefinitely. The first ferry had arrived on scene within about three minutes of the accident, and the other six within ten minutes.

A New York Fire Department rescue boat arrived within eight minutes, followed by two coast guard craft nine minutes later. Video footage showed all of the A320's occupants were rescued within about twenty minutes of the ditching. Early on, a helicopter arrived on the scene but pulled back so that its downdraft would not blow people off the wings—consequently, a frogman had to jump bravely from a much greater height than usual to help a woman in difficulty in the water.

Finally, the rescuers saved everyone, with only five people having what are classed as serious injuries:

The flight attendant who had been at the rear and who did not notice a gash in her leg extending down to the muscle until rescued; A passenger with a fracture of the small ossified extension to the lower part of the sternum; A passenger with hypothermia, kept in hospital for two days; And two passengers with a fractured shoulder who did not initially go to hospital but who in post-accident interviews had medical records proving it.

The Investigation

The investigators were bound to review Sully's decisions and carry out simulator what-if tests to see whether he could have made it back to LaGuardia. In fact, some pilots reenacting the event on the simulator succeeded in doing so by immediately turning back, but none could when thinking time was added in. The idea of factoring in the thirty-five seconds the pilots needed to assess the situation and work out the best course of action came from the investigators and not from Sully.

Even if it had been just about possible to make it back to the airport, would it have been sensible to take the risk when unsure? The investigators concluded Sully made the right decision.

One of the best books on the whole affair is *Fly by Wire: The Geese, The Glide, the "Miracle" on The Hudson*, by William Langewiesche, who not only writes beautifully but, even more importantly, researches his topics in depth.

He describes that public hearing at the NTSB offices at L'Enfant Plaza, in Washington, DC, six months after the event as a missed opportunity, with many questioners either pulling their punches or basking in the glory of the hero, asking leading questions to show themselves or their organizations in the best possible light.

Representatives from Airbus were, on the other hand, chomping at the bit, frustrated that no attempt was made to highlight the fact that their sophisticated Airbus flight control system, which did most of the actual flying and did not allow the A320 to stall, deserved some of the praise.

Richard de Crespigny, the captain of a Qantas Airbus 380 that he brought safely back to Singapore after it was crippled by an uncontained engine disintegration, was full of praise for his aircraft, unlike Sully, who said nothing, perhaps because it was America and he had been told by his various handlers to be guarded in his remarks.

The NTSB made many recommendations, most of which have been virtually ignored, perhaps because such events are a rarity, though the NTSB points out that many airports have stretches of water close by.

Sully the Movie and TV Documentaries

The movie *Sully*, with Tom Hanks as a very credible and likeable Sully, proved a big box office hit in the US and abroad, in great part by making the hero look even more heroic, at the expense of the NTSB investigators.

Unlike the gripping movie *Apollo 13*, where the high drama lasted three days as the capsule with the three astronauts circled the moon, this incident lasted a mere three minutes from the moment of the bird strike to coming down safely on the water.

Therefore, to hold cinemagoers' interest, the filmmakers introduced scenes showing Sully imagining his aircraft hitting Midtown buildings in 9/11 style, and more disconcertingly created a false scenario in which Sully and Skiles are portrayed as victims of a drawn-out NTSB witch hunt, the dramatic finale being that public hearing at the NTSB, at which Sully pulls a cat out of a bag to dramatically prove for all to see that the callous investigators were totally wrong because they had forgotten to factor in "thinking time." In fact, as said, it was the NTSB's idea to factor it in and say he could not have got back to LaGuardia and had indeed acted correctly.

For balance, one should perhaps see the gripping *Air Crash Investigation* TV series, where the honorable NTSB investigators figure personally. Also, the excellent documentary *Miracle of the Hudson Plane Crash*, broadcast in the UK by Channel 4 in February 2009, has good explanations, actual footage, and interviews with the passengers and rescuers, and shows just how difficult the rescue from the icy water was, since the ferries first on the scene were not designed to pluck people out of water or from life rafts, nor retrieve them from aircraft wings—Sully told them to concentrate on those on the wings, as the life rafts could stay afloat indefinitely. Also, everyone survived despite the floating escape chutes not automatically separating from the fuselage and potentially being dragged down by the sinking A320— one of the crew on a rescue craft provided a knife to cut one free.

An Imaginary Father's Response

Let us suppose the incident had occurred other than in full view in New York City and the public had not yet been told the details.

A proud father not wanting to boast of his son's unseen exploit might well have replied to a journalist, "Yes, the boy did well. He not only got them down safely but went through the cabin making quite sure no one remained. I do wonder, though, how many other pilots could have done that."

Patrick Smith, in his bestseller *Pilot Confidential*, says that in many respects landing on the calm Hudson was akin to landing on a twelve-mile-long runway and did not require exceptional piloting abilities.

Good Judgment

Great airmanship includes good judgment. Of prime importance was Sully's in that respect; firstly, in restarting the auxiliary power unit so the Airbus computer could fly the aircraft optimally, all the while providing full instrument displays, and secondly, in deciding not to attempt to reach an airport, which could have meant coming down on buildings, killing all on board together with many on the ground.

Even so, saving *every* single soul on board was contingent on there being a long, straight stretch of smooth water within gliding range, rescue craft three minutes away from the spot where they would logically touch down, and—what was most unusual for an overland domestic flight—the aircraft having life rafts and life vests.

There has been argument between the two esteemed authors already mentioned in this piece, with William Langewiesche saying the A320's computer was the real hero, and Patrick Smith endorsed by others critical of fly-by-wire systems, such as on the A320, where the pilots tell the computer what they want to do, and the computer decides whether it is possible. The latter say the computer has a mind of its own, and that in this case it prevented the aircraft flaring, which resulted in it hitting the water much too hard. They even cite the A320 that came down on trees at Habsheim Air Show, as described in Chapter 17 (see Part 2), allegedly because the computer would not let it climb. They fail to point out that in both cases the computer would not let it climb because the pilots were flying it too slowly to do so, and that a stall could have been worse.

Sully's actual maneuvering of the aircraft—the thing for which, understandably, the public hold him in such high esteem—was the area where he performed well but not perfectly or exceptionally. He let his airspeed fall too low and thus was unable to make an effective flare to break the excessive sink rate, which ultimately resulted in the panels under the tail section breaking and letting in water and the shock injuring the flight attendant sitting there.

The NTSB investigators attributed this failure to maintain airspeed to tunnel vision brought about by lack of time, stress, work overload, the distractions of various alarms, the off-putting sight of skyscrapers alongside, and concentrating on maneuvering the aircraft, and other audible warnings being prioritized over airspeed warnings at that low height.

They pointed out that without thrust from the engines, it would be extremely difficult for any pilot to achieve the recommended ditching speeds, assuming he or she knew them. However, Sully did strike the water with the wings virtually level, and at such a nose-up angle that the aircraft did not spin, cartwheel, or break up, say due to an engine or wingtip nicking the water. He did well enough, but other than keeping his nerve while performing that maneuver, he probably did not need the full panoply of talents honed from the age of three onwards extolled in his autobiography.

With the rear of the aircraft damaged and icy water coming in, perhaps the real "miracle" was the rescue, with not a single fatality thanks to the diligence of so many—boatmen, helicopter men, not forgetting Sully, who checked so thoroughly that everyone was out and gave advice and assistance to those in difficulty. This was also thanks to the cabin crew, all with twenty if not thirty years' experience, showing there is something to be said for that. Admittedly, an average domestic flight might well have had passengers with impaired mobility and made their task more difficult.

One of the many lessons noted by the NTSB investigators is a little chilling for those of us confined in seats so close to the one in front that in adopting the brace position we cannot bend fully over and grab our ankles, and instead have to press on the top of the back of the seat in front with our hands or arms. Two female passengers so doing suffered a shoulder fracture.

A man generously took charge of the baby a mother was carrying on her lap, but had the deceleration been far greater he might not have been able to save it as he did. Babies and infants in arms should ideally have their own seats and restraints; however, that might mean people unable to afford the extra seat would travel by road, which is far more dangerous.

One gratifying endnote is that the passengers who risked the lives of their fellow passengers and cabin crew by bringing their luggage with them lost it in the river, while those that did not got it returned.

One cannot take away Sully's achievement. Just imagine the gut-wrenching feeling he had to overcome on finding himself engineless over a packed metropolis with no height to play with.

Interestingly, Richard de Crespigny in his new book *Fly!* notes that Sully still sees room for improvement in the way people in high-risk occupations such as aviation are trained, and quotes him as saying, "In some ways, I might have been better prepared for Flight 1549 earlier in my career, while still a fighter pilot, perhaps. In that part of my career, I had more frequent equipment failures that I dealt with on a regular basis, and we were always operating closer to the limits in nearly every way. But airline flying is different. While by no means complacent, I had been flying well within the boundaries for many years in an environment where I was—fortunately, of course—not *challenged in any significant way.*"

Indeed, some crashes described in this book would not have occurred had there been better training to enable airline pilots to cope with the startle effect and the unexpected.

Comparison with Ditching of Ethiopian Airliner

The media immediately contrasted Sully's ditching and its perfect outcome with the imperfect one by Captain Leul Abate, the Ethiopian Airlines pilot who ditched his 767 off a beach, with one wing snagging the water and the aircraft spinning around before breaking up, with many lives lost. (A number of passengers were trapped due to premature inflation of their life vests causing them to float upward in the water-filled cabin.)

[Described earlier in this chapter.]

However, they are not comparable:

1. Abate was coming down in the sea with waves;

2. A hijacker was grabbing at the controls;

3. With no fuel left, electrical power was only being provided by the ram air turbine (RAT), a wind-driven generator;

4. With only minimal electric power for the most basic instruments and controls, he could not use any flap and was therefore traveling much too fast, with the aircraft difficult to control.

However, like Sully he did well to come down somewhere where boats could come to the rescue of survivors.

A Very Close-run Thing

Only when one looks closely at the photos of the occupants of the A320 perched precariously on its wings does one realize what a close-run thing it was. The aircraft could have sunk deeper; there could have been jostling, with people falling into the water and dragging others with them.

Again, Sully did great—twice going up and down the cabin to check everyone was out and telling rescuers to first save those on the wings. But had the bird strike occurred a little earlier, with the aircraft not quite so high, he would not have been able to skirt the George Washington Bridge and come down at a shallow angle on the Hudson, let alone at a point where rescue craft were at hand.

It was a miracle—call it what you like—that Sully's feat was capped by the perfect rescue, thanks to an almost unbelievable combination of factors and, not least, diligence on the part of the rescuers—and nothing went seriously wrong, as it so easily could have.

---

[1] Aircraft are handled by the "tower" (local controller (LC)) at takeoff. Once aloft, they are soon handed over to Terminal Radar Approach Control (TRACOM), which controls flights up to a height of 18,000 feet and a range of say 50 miles. Very often TRACOM is called Approach or Departure (control). Here we are talking about "New York TRACOM LaGuardia Departure."

Chapter 2
LOSS OF POWER
OVER LAND

Conscientious Crew Forget How Much Fuel Left (Portland, 1978)

An absurd accident that led to great improvements

> Following this accident United Airlines introduced a new training concept called CRM or Crew Resource Management. Now universally applied, even in medicine.
>
> United Airlines Flight 173, December 28, 1978

On December 28, 1978, a United Airlines McDonnell Douglas DC-8 with the flight number 173 was approaching Portland Airport in Oregon. The 189 people on board included the captain, the first officer, a flight engineer, a deadheading captain two weeks from retirement, and four cabin attendants. There were six infants. ETA was 17:15.

On leaving the gate at the previous stopover, there had been enough fuel for the two-hour, twenty-six-minute leg to Portland, with an additional forty-five-minute fuel reserve to meet FAA requirements and a further approximately twenty-minute fuel reserve to meet company contingency requirements. Portland Approach Control had given them clearance to make a straight-in landing on Runway 28, so they should have been landing with their fuel reserve of just over an hour intact.

As they descended through six thousand feet with the runway in sight, the first officer, who was the pilot flying (PF), requested fifteen degrees of flap and the lowering of the landing gear. The captain extended the flaps to fifteen degrees and initiated the lowering of the landing gear, which to his surprise dropped down with an unusual thump and more quickly than usual. The captain said the first officer had noticed a simultaneous yaw to the right.

The jolt was even more noticeable to the flight attendants and passengers farther back in the aircraft. More disconcertingly, one of the landing gear indicator lights failed to show green, presenting the crew with the worrying possibility that the right-hand landing gear assembly was not properly down and locked.

Unaware of any such problem, Portland Approach told them to switch to the Portland Tower frequency for the actual landing. UA173 declined, saying they had a "gear problem" and wanted to stay with approach, maintaining a height of five thousand feet and a speed of 170 knots. According to AVweb.com, one of the approach controllers in question said as recently as 1998/9 that the controller gave the captain the option of holding at six thousand feet over the Laker outer compass locator until he sorted out the problem. From there he could have made a dead-stick landing at any time onto either runway, but instead he opted to orbit twenty miles or so southeast of the airport.

Approach agreed to this request to orbit, telling them to turn left onto a heading of two hundred degrees to take them away from the airport and out of the path of any other incoming aircraft.

They carried out various checks, even contacting the company's San Francisco Maintenance Control Center, who could not think of anything further. The captain then briefed the senior flight attendant about getting ready for an emergency landing and possible evacuation but did not give her a deadline or suggest any state of urgency. (He later said he assumed it would take ten or fifteen minutes, and that final preparations could be carried out as they came in to land.)

At that time, all three aircrew were fully aware of the fuel situation, since at 17:46:52 the flight engineer replied to the first officer that they had five thousand pounds of fuel left. Not only did the first officer acknowledge this, he immediately asked the captain,

What's the fuel show now?

The captain replied,

Five.

The first officer duly repeated,

Five.

Further confirmation that there was only about five thousand pounds of fuel left was given by the fact that the inboard fuel pump lamps started to blink, as they are meant to do if the fuel level falls below five thousand pounds. The aircraft was about thirteen nautical miles south of the airport and heading away from it.

With not much time before the fuel would run out, they yet again discussed the status of the landing gear, before being interrupted by a course change and advisory from approach control.

17:50:20 Captain to flight engineer:
Give us a current card on weight. Figure about another fifteen minutes.

Flight engineer:
Fifteen minutes?

Captain:
Yeah, give us three or four thousand pounds on top of zero fuel weight.

Flight engineer:
Not enough. Fifteen minutes is gonna . . . really run us low on fuel here.

The two pilots then busied themselves with preparations for landing, while the flight engineer replied to questions from the company representative at Portland about the fuel load on landing and the number of passengers. Finally, the flight engineer asked the captain whether he could inform the company representative that they would be landing at "five after." The captain said, "Yeah."

At 17:55:04 the flight engineer reported completion of the approach descent check. When the first officer, at 17:56:53, asked about how much fuel he had, the flight engineer replied that four thousand pounds remained—one thousand pounds in each tank. The captain then sent the flight engineer to the passenger cabin "to kinda see how things are going." In his absence, the captain and first officer discussed the importance of giving the flight attendants time to prepare, what cockpit procedures would be required in the event of an emergency evacuation, and finally whether the brake antiskid devices would be working.

At 18:01:12, Portland Approach put them on another orbit.

United 173 heavy turn left, heading one niner five.

By complying with those instructions to orbit instead of requesting immediate clearance to proceed with the landing in accordance with the initial timetable, the first officer—with the captain's apparent acquiescence—sealed the fate of the aircraft.

At 18:01:34, the flight engineer returned to the flight deck with the news that everything would be ready in another two or three minutes. He and the captain briefly discussed the mood and state of the passengers.

18:02:22 Flight engineer:

We got about three on the fuel and that's it.

Captain:

Okay. On touchdown, if the gear folds or something really jumps the track, get those boost pumps off so that . . . you might even get the valves open.

At 18:02:44, approach control, no doubt surprised that the whole affair was taking so long, asked to be appraised of the situation and was told by the first officer that they still had an indication of a landing gear abnormality, they expected to land in about five minutes, and would need emergency services standing by. At 18:03:14, with the aircraft about eight nautical miles south of the airport and heading away from it, Portland Approach told them to advise when they would like to begin their approach.

The captain replied,

> They've about finished in the cabin. I'd guess about
> another three, four, five minutes.

As is customary for a possible emergency landing, Portland Approach asked for a final confirmation as to the number of souls on board and the amount of fuel remaining.

The flight crew spent the next two and half minutes discussing technical matters. They wondered whether the horn that warns pilots if they are landing without the landing gear locked down might not be a helpful indication of its true status. They also wondered whether the tripping of the landing gear circuit breakers might mean the spoilers and antiskid brakes would not deploy automatically.

The senior flight attendant came back to the flight deck to report that she thought they were ready, with the aircraft by then about seventeen nautical miles south of the airport and still heading away from it. After talking to her for about a half minute and going into detail about whether able-bodied people were by the exits, and noting the fact that the off-duty captain would be in the first row of coach behind the galley, the captain said to her:

> Okay. We're going to go in now. We should be landing
> in about five minutes.

It was 18:06:40, and they were nineteen nautical miles south-southwest of the airport and still heading *away* from it.

Before the flight attendant could answer, the flight engineer or the first officer interjected:

I think you lost number four, buddy, you . . .

Flight attendant:

Okay, I'll make the five-minute announcement. I'll go. I'm sitting down now.

First officer to flight engineer:

Better get some cross feeds open there or something!

Flight engineer:

Okay!

"All righty," said the flight attendant on starting to make her way back to the passenger cabins.

At 18:06:46, the first officer twice told the captain they were going to lose an engine. The captain twice replied, "Why?" to which the first officer each time replied, "Fuel." They both told the flight engineer to open the cross feeds, and there seemed to be some confusion as to how much fuel they had.

At 18:07:06, the first officer declared the engine had flamed out. At 18:07:12, almost an hour after declining their initial clearance to make a landing approach, the captain finally asked for it again. The controller accordingly gave him an initial heading vector of 010 degrees, to which they turned, and they were again nineteen nautical miles south-southwest of the airport.

18:07:27 Flight engineer

We're going to lose number three in a minute too.

The crew tried to see if they could keep the engines going by opening cross feeds.

18:10:47 Approach:

Eighteen flying miles from the field.

18:12:43 Approach:

Twelve flying miles from the field.

The flight engineer declared they had just lost two engines, "One and two."

18:13:29 Approach:

Eight or nine flying miles from the field.

18:13:38 Captain:

They're all going. We can't make Troutdale [a nearer general aviation airport].

18:13:43 First officer:

We can't make anything!

The captain then told him to declare a Mayday. The first officer did so, ending his transmission to the tower with the words:

We're going down. We're not going to be able to reach the airport.

The captain later said that in the minute or so he could remain in the air there were few options, and no good ones. Congestion due to rush-hour traffic would make landing on the highway along the bank of the Columbia River a disastrous proposition, and icy water in the fast-moving river itself would certainly result in many fatalities, even should he be successful in ditching there in the darkness. He therefore opted to bring the aircraft down in a wooded area with no visible lights about six nautical miles east-southeast of the airport.

His skill no doubt helped keep casualties to a minimum.

Initial impacts were with trees, before the aircraft destroyed two fortunately unoccupied homes. Just before the aircraft came to a halt almost five hundred meters from the point of initial impact with the first tree, the vertical stabilizer on the tail snagged some high-tension electric transmission lines, and this encounter no doubt helped bring the aircraft to a final halt. An outbreak of fire, earlier so much feared by the crew, did not occur, since there was no fuel left. A tree penetrating the fuselage near the flight engineer's position caused some fatalities back from there.

Remarkably, "only" 8 passengers and 2 crew (the flight engineer and the senior flight attendant, who was said to have saved lives by preparing so well for the possible emergency evacuation) were killed. A further 21 passengers and 2 crew members incurred serious injuries. Out of the 189 persons on board, 158 escaped relatively unscathed.

The passengers did not receive any warning from the aircrew that the aircraft was coming down and initially thought they were landing at the airport. After they started striking the trees, a flight attendant shouted out, "Hold your ankles!"

The Inquiry

The inquiry revealed that a fault due to corrosion in part of the landing gear mechanism caused one set of wheels to free-fall down into place rather than sink down gently. The temporary imbalance in drag (one set of wheels came down earlier than the other) produced the yaw noticed by the first officer.

Furthermore, in the process of dropping down so sharply into place, the gear damaged the micro-switches used to show whether it was fully down and locked. In fact, the aircraft could have landed safely at any time.

The inquiry concluded that the crew, having become so absorbed in trying to solve the landing gear problem and thinking about all the possible consequences, failed properly to consider the fuel consumption rate. However, they did note that when asked about the fuel they would have if they landed as planned (at five past the hour), the flight engineer had said, "Fifteen minutes is gonna . . . really run us low on fuel here!"

For the hour they were orbiting, the captain was considering every eventuality, including the mental state of the passengers, in detail. He even sought to arrange for the San Francisco Maintenance Office to handle certain procedures to avoid the risk of bad local publicity.

The incident revealed the need for formal policies and programs to ensure aircrew function well as a team, with each having defined complementary duties rather than everyone focusing on the same detail. Now called "Crew Resource Management" (CRM).

Miscalculation Meant Only Half the Fuel Loaded (Gimli, 1983)

Superlative piloting technique saved the day

> Considering there are relatively few instances of airliners, such as Piché's, gliding long distances to a safe landing, it is surprising that another Canada-registered one had featured eighteen years before in a similar feat, but over land.
>
> Air Canada Flight 143, July 23, 1983

Captain Bob Pearson and First Officer Quintal were flying their sophisticated Air Canada Boeing 767 between Ottawa and Edmonton when it ran out of fuel out of gliding range to a major airport.

They had set off with their fuel gauges not working, and the flight management computer (FMC) was calculating the amount of fuel in the tanks by deducting the amount consumed by the engines from the amount measured by dipsticks on departure. Thus, the amount shown depended on correctly knowing the amount of fuel initially in the tanks.

Regardless of whatever the FMC said, they should have had no need to worry, as the dipstick checks at Montreal and then Ottawa had shown they had ample fuel for the 3,574-kilometer leg to Edmonton and would still have the required reserves.

Just over halfway, with the readout from the FMC indicating several tons of fuel left, a beeping sound drew the relaxing pilots' attention to low pressure in one of the two fuel pumps feeding the left engine. Soon afterward the instruments indicated low pressure in the other pump. Was it a computer glitch or faulty sensors? However, the aircraft was virtually new, and to have two pumps, or their pressure sensors, fail was troubling enough for Pearson to decide to divert to the nearest appropriate airport, which was Winnipeg.

Still at forty-one thousand feet, they throttled back the engines to begin descent into Winnipeg, some 120 nautical miles away.

Shortly afterward the displays warned of a similar low fuel-pump pressure situation for both pumps feeding the engine on the opposite side. For so many pumps to be affected simultaneously was a sure sign of a fuel problem, and their fears were confirmed when only a few minutes later the number one engine flamed out, followed three minutes later by the number two engine.

Normally, the fuel measurement system would have given a warning once the fuel level fell to two tons, giving them more than adequate time (over land) to make an emergency landing under power. But of course, that was not working.

They were by then down to twenty-five thousand feet, with still sixty-five nautical miles to go to Winnipeg. As in the case of Piché's aircraft, a small RAT (ram air turbine) had dropped down from the underside of the aircraft to provide just enough power for very basic flying controls and instruments. The once-sophisticated screens were blank, and all they had was the artificial horizon, airspeed indicator, altimeter, and a magnetic compass, which was difficult to read because, unlike the usual gyrocompass, it was not stable.

With no vertical speed indicator, judging the optimum glide path was exceedingly difficult, and amid his other tasks, the first officer had to get the Winnipeg controller to constantly give the distance remaining to Winnipeg and try to work it out from tables.

With them down to 10,000 feet and descending to 9,500 feet, the distance remaining was forty-five nautical miles. They were losing height faster than expected, and at that rate all hope of making Winnipeg had gone. The situation was desperate.

Just as the captain was about to ask Winnipeg for anything nearer, the first officer suggested they try Gimli Air Force Base, where he had been temporarily stationed during his military service. He knew it had two runways of sufficient length. Reassuringly, air traffic control informed them Gimli was only twelve nautical miles from their location.

The air traffic controller guided them toward Gimli but with some difficulty, as not being operational, the field itself was not shown on the charts. The captain was informed of this but told light aircraft were using the *right-hand* runway. The controller could not guarantee the runway would be clear.

They did not want to lose too much height before being sure they could identify the Gimli base, and the trouble was that although the first officer knew the general area, he could not be sure exactly where it would be. When he finally did sight it, they were much too high, posing the problem of how to lose both height and speed in the distance that remained without the help of flaps or air brakes.

By a lucky coincidence, Captain Pearson happened to be an experienced glider pilot. With no air brakes, he had to resort to a series of difficult sideslips and yaws, with the ailerons sending the aircraft one way and the rudder the opposite way to provide a braking effect that only a glider pilot could execute, he brought the speed and height down to a reasonable degree; and with the runway ahead, told the first officer to lower the landing gear.

In the dusk, they could only see one clearly defined, whitish runway ahead and assumed incorrectly it must be the right-hand one on which they planned to land. Unknowingly, they were lining up with the disused left-hand runway, which that weekend was being used as a racing car circuit, with a strip down the middle and the cars going down one side and up the other.

The first officer duly selected "Landing Gear Down," but nothing happened. Frantically, he searched in the manual to see how to let the wheels fall just by gravity but could not find the explanation—actually, and logically, in the hydraulics section—because the index failed to mention it. He then tried the alternative gear extension switch and, with a sigh of relief, heard the wheels drop down. To his consternation there was no green light to confirm the nose wheel had locked.

To slow the aircraft and lose more height the captain had to bank the aircraft steeply and apply rudder to make it fly crabwise, frightening the passengers looking straight down at astonished people on a golf course.

Even so, coming in fifty knots faster than normal, he made a perfect landing on the wrong runway, only to find there were people, including children, on it.

Luckily, the last race of the day had just finished, and all were congregated at the far end. Also, having caught sight of the silent aircraft coming in, drivers rushed to move their cars, while others screamed at a boy riding up and down the runway, quite oblivious to what was happening. Luckily, the aircraft missed him.

The captain applied the brakes as hard as possible, and as the aircraft slowed, the unlocked nose-wheel assembly collapsed to produce a shower of sparks. The failure of the front wheel was a blessing in disguise, as it helped stop the aircraft just short of a group of very surprised adults and children.

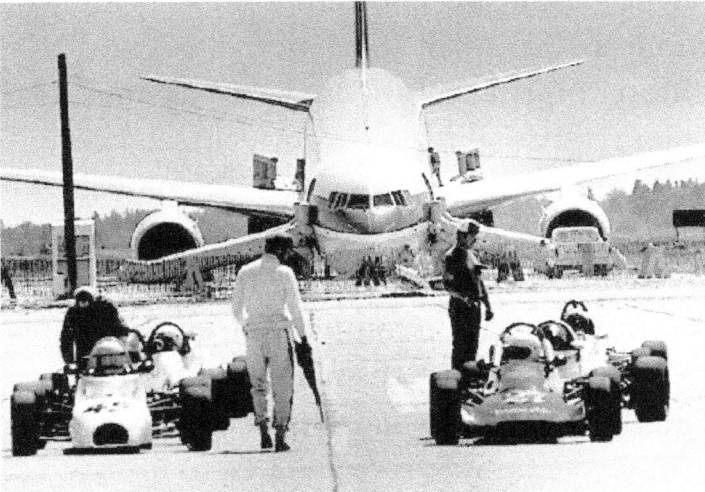

With the collapse of the nose-wheel assembly, the aircraft had tilted forward with the tail high up in the air, making the chutes at the rear too steep to use safely.

However, with relatively few passengers on board, all were able to exit easily and safely from the front. Again, with no fuel there was little likelihood of a major fire, and fire extinguishers from the race organizers ensured smoke coming from the front did not develop into a serious fire.

As usual a series of failures and misunderstandings were responsible for this ridiculous near disaster.

There are so many little factors that not every reader will want to read this next part in full:

Multiple Causes

1. Noncompliance with the MEL, minimum equipment list.
    For safety reasons, essential systems in aircraft are in duplicate, triplicate, and sometimes quadruplicate.
    In addition, some items are not safety critical, in the sense that they do not significantly affect safety.
    Therefore, for every aircraft there is a MEL showing what systems or items must be working. The pilots run through this list before every flight and check their aircraft meets minimum requirements before setting out, even though the maintenance personnel will have verified this before handing over.

    Sometimes there may be a special-case MEL with conditions attached to it. For instance, when maintenance staff in Tokyo found a faulty engine on a 747 that could not be easily or cheaply repaired there, the airline, British Airways, decided to have it repaired in London. It was able to fly the aircraft back to London on three engines on the condition that there were no passengers and it had an extra pilot, who would have to come from London to assist. A three-engine ferry flight must have a specially trained captain, as improper application of asymmetric power can be disastrous.

Many of the provisions in the MEL are obvious and apply to similar aircraft, but others are specific to a particular aircraft type. When a new aircraft is developed, the aircraft manufacturer issues a MEL, which the airline and manufacturer update. The newly developed and sophisticated Boeing 767 (with screens replacing many traditional dials) was a completely new aircraft for Air Canada, so the MEL was not definitive. With so many revisions, pilots often had to check with maintenance management to be sure of what was permissible.

When Pearson arrived at Montreal Airport with First Officer Quintal, they met the incoming captain, Captain Weir, and naturally discussed the condition of the aircraft. Weir said there was a problem with the fuel gauges and went on to mention the fact that they had once blanked out. Weir himself had misunderstood the technician in Edmonton, who had said they had blanked out coming in from Toronto several weeks earlier; Weir thought he meant that they had blanked on the flight that had just come in from Toronto. Anyway, Captain

Pearson believed the aircraft he was to take over had come in with all the fuel gauges blanked out and that it would be reasonable to carry on likewise, especially as the new part was waiting in Edmonton, their destination.

It would have been difficult for Pearson to refuse to fly an aircraft that he thought other captains had deemed acceptable, and especially so when maintenance had confirmed that complying with the MEL did not pose a problem. In fact, the other captains had flown the aircraft with the fuel gauges working with input from just one processor channel, which satisfied the MEL, provided ground staff carried out a dipstick check as well. Maintenance was wrong to say departing with **none** of the fuel gauges working complied with the MEL.

2. The Technical Fault

Much earlier the technician in Edmonton had found that the entire fuel gauge system blanked out when one of the digital processor channels failed. Failure of one element in a two-channel fuel indication system should not have crippled the entire system. However, poor design (not by Boeing) meant there was not enough power when one side failed, and this accounted for the whole system going blank from time to time, because of a fickle connection due to cold soldering in the right-hand channel.

Any car owner knows how difficult it is to find an intermittent fault, as it is never there when you are looking for it. It can also lure the user into a sense of false security, as things may revert to normal for a long time, only for a failure to occur when there is a temperature or pressure change or when there is turbulence. This is why the faulty part in Pearson's aircraft was not repaired earlier.

3. Misunderstandings: Language

The qualified technician in Edmonton found he could get the fuel gauges to work by isolating the defective processor channel. He therefore switched off that channel and agreed with maintenance that the aircraft could fly like that while waiting for the spare part, provided a dipstick check was carried out. He left a note on the tripped circuit breaker saying the channel was inoperative. In the maintenance log, he wrote:

SERVICE CHK—FOUND FUEL QTY IND BLANK— FUEL QTY #2 C/B PULLED & TAGGED—FUEL DIP REQD PRIOR TO DEP. SEE MEL.

4. Too Many Cooks

Had no one else stuck their oar in, all would have been well, at least as regards keeping the fuel gauges functioning. Unfortunately, while waiting to dipstick the tanks after refueling in Montreal, a less-qualified technician noticed the pulled circuit breaker with the tag saying, "Not Operational." Though not properly qualified to test the system, he tried resetting the breaker, thus making the fuel gauges go blank. Before he had time to re-pull the breaker and see if that made the gauges work, he was called away to check the tanks using a dipstick. He forgot about it but did remember to put a note in the log:

FUEL QTY IND U/S. SUSPECT PROCESSOR UNIT AT FAULT. NIL STOCK.

He then signed off the maintenance log as satisfactory.

5. Metric Conversion Error

When dealing with fuel volumes, such as when refueling or using a dipstick to check the amount of fuel in a tank, the unit used is the liter. However, weight is what the pilots want to know, as it is so important when flying. For instance, the V takeoff speeds vary according to the gross weight of the aircraft.

As Stanley Stewart says in his excellent account in *Emergency: Crisis on The Flightdeck*, the technician was referring to the fuel indicators going blank during the check, but that would not be clear from the text. Of course, the technician's "SEE MEL" supposedly, but not obviously, restated the need to have a dipstick check, as well as one processor channel working.

Up to that time the unit used to express weight at the airline had been pounds. Like many countries other than the United States, Canada was changing over to the metric system, and the 767 was the first aircraft type in the Air Canada fleet to have the fuel weight expressed in kilograms rather than pounds.

Everyone dealing with that 767 knew the weight of the fuel had to be expressed in kilograms, but in converting liters to kilograms they all used or copied the wrong conversion factor. Any kid educated at school in the metric system would have known that one liter of water weighs one kilogram and would realize that with kerosene being slightly lighter than water, one would have to use a conversion factor of slightly less than one (actually 0.8). Instead, they used the conversion factor for converting liters to pounds, which is 1.77. As a result, they only had some ten tonnes (metric tons) of fuel in the tanks and imagined they had twenty-two, and that was the figure programmed into the FMC which was calculating the amount of fuel remaining by deducting the amount burned from that.

On checking the calculations, Captain Pearson, not expecting an error of that nature, failed to notice the use of the wrong conversion factor.

Conclusion

This incident was the result of many errors and failures. As renowned safety academic, Professor Reason, says, with the best will in the world it is impossible to prevent all errors, and the important thing is finding ways to cope with them. Failure to follow the MEL and the bad design of the overall fuel processor system, which allowed failure of one part to cripple the entire system, would seem to be key errors.

Badly relayed information and cryptic technical logs also played a significant part. Unfamiliarity with weight and volume conversions was also a factor, meaning the obvious mistake was not realized.

A Piloting Feat

Captain Pearson's landing on that short landing strip, with the need to use his glider-flying skills to lose so much height and attenuate airspeed, represented a remarkable feat. However, if the day's motor-racing events had not just finished it would have been a different story.

TACA Deadstick Landing on Grass Levee (New Orleans, 1988)

Great feat of airmanship, by a captain with one eye

> The captain was going to ditch in the water but at the last moment saw a relatively flat grass levee on the bank. He landed there with no loss of life despite having only one eye.
>
> TACA Flight 110, May 24, 1988

T ACA, a small airline based in El Salvador and founded in 1931, was so proud of its brand-new Boeing 737-3 that when Flight 110 encountered severe hail, the pilots' first concern was that it might damage the paintwork.

The flight had taken off in fine weather from Belize City with thirty-eight passengers and seven crew, but on crossing over the Gulf of Mexico, known for its fickle weather, the weather radar showed storms ahead. The pilots tried to skirt the parts shown in red, with the heaviest rain, and keep to the areas shown in green and yellow, where the rain would be less intense.

Though the captain, Carlos Dardano, and second officer, Dionisio Lopez, were relatively young, they were very experienced. Sitting in the jump seat was a senior training pilot, who had come along get some experience of being on a new 737. As they approached their destination, New Orleans, they commenced their descent from thirty-five thousand feet.

On their weather radar they saw a gap, shown in green and yellow areas, with red ones on either side ahead, and entered the cloud at thirty thousand feet, having turned on the engine anti-icing and engine auto-ignition so that an engine would immediately restart should it flame out.

As they descended lower and lower, they were surprised at the amount of rain, turbulence, and especially hail, despite it not having been displayed as red on their radar. Since hail is dry, it does not show up properly on radar.

At sixteen thousand feet, both engines flamed out almost simultaneously, leaving them gliding without even electrical power for their instruments, other than a few key ones with battery backup. Their radio was out, so they could not communicate with air traffic control (ATC).

They started the auxiliary power unit (APU) in the tail, but that took time to power up, at which point, with electricity for their communications, they could discuss possible landing places with ATC. They were low in dense air and had the engines windmilling at the right speed for restarting but were unsuccessful.

Getting desperate, they finally managed to restart them using the engine starters with electric power supplied by the APU. Sighing with relief, they prematurely informed ATC they no longer needed to come down immediately and would continue to New Orleans. ATC duly gave them the course for that. However, the engines were not producing any meaningful thrust. Worse, when the pilots opened the throttles to push more fuel in, the engines overheated to the point where it was obvious they would catch fire or explode, which meant they had to be shut down immediately and definitively.

The overheating was because it was a hot start—that is, excess fuel in the engine was catching fire. The pilots cannot be blamed, because at such a low height they could not take their time and allow it to bleed away.

They were at three thousand feet with just three minutes left. They had dismissed the suggestion by ATC of coming down on a highway, for, with vehicles on it, the maneuver would be fraught with danger, both for those in the aircraft and on the ground. The only serious option was to ditch in one of the wide waterways. One lay straight ahead, and the captain aimed to ditch near the bank.

Then, as they came down below two thousand feet, copilot Lopez pointed out the grass-covered levee to the side on the right. Perhaps to get a clearer view and make sure the ground there was as flat and obstacle-free as it appeared, Captain Dardano may have continued to aim for the water before doing a deft sideslip to line up with the levee.

Passing over the wall at the near end, he touched down perfectly and with no reverse thrust to help bring the thirty-seven-ton airliner to a halt by delicate application of the brakes to prevent it skidding out of control. There was no fire and all on board evacuated safely via the slides, with only one very minor injury.

A truly remarkable feat.

But how could the almost brand new 737 be retrieved. Would it have to be taken to pieces?

Finally, with one engine completely replaced and the other repaired, and things removed to reduce weight, two test pilots flew the aircraft, with just enough fuel to reach the airport, off the levee.

CFM56 Engine Used Worldwide

There was great concern, for the CFM56 engine was used in many aircraft worldwide in addition to the ubiquitous 737. The fact that such a reliable engine could in certain circumstances flame out in a storm, with subsequent problems when restarted, was very troubling.

The investigators had the engine maker redo the acceptance tests, but no matter how much water they injected, they could not get the engines to stop.

They then studied the readings on the TACA cockpit data recorder more closely and noticed that when the engines flamed out the aircraft was beginning its descent into New Orleans under low power. The test was therefore repeated at low power settings and showed that a large amount of water in the core—simulating the presence of hail—did make it flame out.

Minor modifications were made to CFM56 engines, including better pathways to bleed away water, reshaping fan blades to help divert small hail particles from the core, and a sensor to make the ignitors fire automatically in heavy rain or hail.

Avianca 52 Copilot Failed to Say "Emergency" (New York, 1990)

Did not tell controller it was their last chance to land

> The survivors and relatives of those who died when
> Avianca Flight 52 ran out of fuel while attempting to land
> at New York's JFK airport were incensed when reminded
> the official inquiry attributed the accident almost entirely
> to the first officer's failure to use the term "emergency" in
> his radio transmissions to air traffic control.
>
> Avianca Flight 52, January 25, 1990

The lights in the passenger cabin of the Colombian Avianca Boeing 707 flickered as the fuel supply to the engines became erratic. With so little fuel left, no measure could save them other than coming down on a runway or flat, open space. However, JFK airport was fifteen miles away, and the hilly ground of the affluent residential district of Cove Neck, on Long Island, lay ahead.

A few seconds later the engines fell silent, leaving only the rustle of the wind against the fuselage, soon to be drowned out by the screams and exclamations of the passengers realizing they might be facing their maker.

How, in what one would imagine to be one of the most sophisticated air traffic control (ATC) zones in the world, could the pilots and passengers of Avianca Flight 52 find themselves in such a predicament?

It was due to what with hindsight was a whole series of missed opportunities to avoid disaster.

The first of these was not diverting to their alternate, Boston, when, on approaching the New York control zone an hour and a half earlier.

Controllers had informed them their wait in the holding pattern would be at least forty-five minutes. The pilots possibly thought the controller was being careful and that the wait would not be very much longer. In fact, they had to hold for seventy-seven minutes.

Then, as the aircraft was subsequently handed over from one controller to another, the first officer, who was handling radio communications, used phrases such as "We're running out of fuel." He evidently thought this clearly indicated their fuel predicament, but he failed to convey the true situation to the controllers, who had perhaps fifty aircraft in the sky, all in a sense running out of fuel and all wanting priority.

If the controllers began letting aircraft that had not declared a real emergency jump the queue, a traffic jam would develop over the airport, perhaps compromising the safety of other aircraft also low on fuel.

Another factor explaining the controllers' apparent lack of probing into Avianca 52's status was that, with the aircraft being handed over successively from controller to controller, none had the time to build up a detailed picture. Aircraft have to be pigeonholed in the controller's mind, and this is particularly so at busy times; for them it is either a normal flight or declared emergency.

When after seventy-seven minutes Flight 52 was allowed to exit the holding pattern (after the crew were asked how much longer they could hold).

It was passed on to the approach controller, who, unaware of their predicament, greeted them as follows:

21:03:11 Approach:

Avianca zero five two heavy, New York Approach, good evening. Fly heading zero six zero.

After acknowledging this, the Avianca flight crew, consisting of the captain, first officer, and flight engineer, agreed on the need, when less than a thousand pounds of fuel remains in any tank, to avoid doing anything, such as raise the nose too much or accelerate violently, that might cause it to slosh to one side, leaving the outlet uncovered.

As the controllers brought them in and gave them course changes, the first officer and flight engineer surmised they were being accommodated and that the controllers were aware of their situation. At no point did they tell the approach controller they were low on fuel, no doubt assuming that the previous controller told him. Apart from the controller telling them to make their speed 160 knots if practical, there is nothing of note from the controller before he hands them over to the tower controller, who greets them:

21:15:23 Tower:

Avianca zero five two heavy, Kennedy Tower, runway two two left. You're number three following seven-two-seven traffic on a, ah, niner mile final.

The tower, finding the more modern aircraft following behind was in danger of catching up with the old Boeing 707, asked Avianca 52 for their airspeed (140 knots) and asked them to increase it by 10 knots, impatiently telling them "Increase! Increase!"

Avianca 52's captain, who was flying the aircraft, seemed to be having some difficulty hearing these exchanges and what the first officer and flight engineer were saying.

They proceeded with the standard prelanding checks and the lowering of the landing gear. Duly cleared to land, they asked for a wind check and were told it was 190 degrees at 20 knots. (The wind speed at their location was apparently of the order of 60 knots, with the difference between that and the 20 knots given to them for the airport representing considerable wind shear.)

The tower, still concerned about the separation from the TWA aircraft behind them, asked for their airspeed again, and on being told it was one four five, asked the TWA aircraft behind if they could match it.

The TWA pilot said:

Okay, we'll do our best.

The Avianca flight was all set for landing but sank a little below the glide slope.

The tower, increasingly concerned about the separation, asked the TWA craft to reduce its final airspeed, if feasible. With the TWA crew saying they could not go slower, the tower asked Avianca 52 to increase theirs by ten knots, but finding they were getting too close, ordered the TWA heavy to turn off to the left and maintain two thousand feet.

The tower then informed American Airlines Flight 40 they had become number two in the landing sequence, behind a 707 (Avianca 52).

It was then, with everything seemingly fine for the landing, that Avianca 52 encountered wind shear two and half nautical miles from the runway. The aircraft sank, with the "Whoop! Whoop! Pull up!" from the ground proximity warning system (GPWS) telling the crew they were in danger of hitting the ground.

To recover, the captain pushed the throttles forward, thus using up much of the remaining fuel. After sinking to the dangerously low height of two hundred feet two miles from the runway, the aircraft finally pulled out of its descent.

Captain:

Where is the runway?

The GPWS repeated:

Whoop! Whoop! Pull up!
Whoop! Whoop! Pull up!
Whoop! Whoop! Pull up!

Captain:

The runway! Where is it?

The automatic "Glide slope!" warning sounded twice.

First officer:

I don't see it! I don't see it!

The captain ordered the raising of the landing gear as they aborted the landing. The glide slope warning sounded twice again, presumably because they were by then above it. The first officer then informed the tower they were executing a missed approach.

It is very likely that the pilots failed to see the runway in the poor visual conditions due to the nose-up attitude of the aircraft at the critical moment as they recovered from the perilous sink rate brought about by the wind shear.

The tower told them to climb and maintain two thousand feet and subsequently asked them to confirm they were making a left turn according to the standard missed landing procedure, exactly as the TWA craft had done just before. The captain then specifically told the first officer to tell the controllers it was an *emergency*. Instead, the first officer simply confirmed to the controller they were executing the left turn as instructed, adding that they were running out of fuel.

First officer to ATC:

> *That's right, to one eight zero on the heading—and, ah, we'll try once again. We're running out of fuel.*

The tower simply said "Okay" and gave the next aircraft, American Airlines Flight 40, clearance to land, adding that a DC-9 had reported wind shear, with a gain and loss of ten knots, from seven hundred feet down to the surface. The Avianca captain once again told his first officer to tell the tower it was an emergency, adding, "Did you tell him?"

First officer replied:

> *Yes, sir. I already advised him.*

This was not strictly true, as the first officer had not used the term "emergency."

In addition, as pointed out by the NTSB investigators, the flight engineer had failed to remind the pilots that to all intents and purposes that had represented their one and only chance to land. This fact should also have been made clear to approach control and the tower lest they order a go-around, such as the one they ordered the TWA aircraft to execute for lack of separation.

Also, even without using the term *"emergency,"* it is difficult to understand why, in the even more desperate situation following the missed approach, the first officer failed to inform the tower they had under ten minutes of fuel left. Some have suggested it was because they were unable to work out a precise figure!

Whether it would have been possible to free up either of JFK's very long 31L or 31R runways and get the Avianca flight far out enough to line up and come in with sufficient fuel remaining is open to question. Performing flying club antics with an airliner would have been difficult enough even in good visibility.

Thus, not realizing the severity of the situation, the tower controller, who was about to hand over to a colleague at the end of his shift, simply handed them over to the approach controller.

The Avianca captain told the first officer to tell approach they didn't have fuel, but the first officer, after automatically acknowledging the order to climb and maintain three thousand feet, reverted to saying, "We are running out of fuel, sir." The controller replied "Okay" and gave them a new heading.

Again, the captain asked the first officer if he had advised ATC they didn't have fuel. He confirmed that he had, adding optimistically, "And he's going to get us back."

The approach controller then gave instructions to two other aircraft. After giving Avianca 52 a new heading, he showed his concern as one can see from the following exchange.

21:26:35 Approach control:

And Avianca zero five two heavy, ah, I'm going to bring you fifteen miles northeast and then bring you back onto the approach. Is that fine with you and your fuel?

21:26:43 First officer:

I guess so. Tha [sic] you very much.

The captain asked what the controller said, but the flight engineer cut in, saying bizarrely, "The guy is angry!"

Approach control continued to give instructions both to them and to other aircraft as if things were normal. At one point, on being asked to climb, they replied in the negative, saying they were running out of fuel. Approach replied, "Okay" and gave a slightly different heading. The controller, knowing they did not have much fuel, evidently wanted to avoid them creeping up on the aircraft in front and having to go around again.

21:31:01 Approach control:

Okay, and you're number two for the approach. I just have to give you enough room so you can make it without, ah, having to come out again.

The first officer acknowledged, and the controller replied, "Thank you, sir." This was hardly the sign of an angry controller, unless said sarcastically, and presumably the controller would be far too busy for such niceties. The controller then dealt with a couple of other aircraft before giving Avianca 52 a thirty-degree change of heading to the left to bring it nearer the heading for the outer marker.

21:32:38 CVR **anomaly**

[hiccup due to fluctuating power supply, no doubt corresponding to flickering of cabin lights.]

21:32:39 Flight engineer:

Flame out! Flame out on engine number four.

21:32:49 Captain:

Show me the runway.

21:32:49 First officer to controller:

Avianca zero five two. We just, ah, lost two engines and, ah, we need priority, please.

The controller then gave them a new heading to intercept the localizer more quickly.

21:32:56 [Sound of engine(s?) spooling down]

The two pilots then talked about setting the instrument landing system. The captain says, "Set the ILS. Let's see."

21:33:04 Approach control:

Avianca zero five two heavy, you're one five miles from the outer marker; maintain two thousand until established on the localizer. Cleared for ILS two two left.

Avianca 52 acknowledged this.

21:33:22 Captain:

Did you select the ILS?

21:33:22 First officer:

It is ready on two.

21:33.24 [End of CVR recording.]

In view of the CVR hiccups when the power supply fluctuated, it is evident that there was no battery backup, and the end of the recording did not correspond with the impact with the ground.

The flight data recorder provided no evidence, because someone had rendered it inoperable by taping back the foil inside. However, examination of the engines at the crash site immediately revealed they had not been rotating under power when the aircraft struck the ground.

Surviving passengers and the only surviving crew member, the leading flight attendant, were able to describe the last moments. Radar records gave useful information about heights and tracks.

According to a witness on the ground, the aircraft dropped silently out of the sky.

Without evidence from the flight data recorder, ascertaining the precise sink rate and forward speed prior to impact was impossible.

Wreckage and Survivors

From the distribution of the debris and the injuries to passengers, it was possible to deduce that the forward speed on impact had not been so great. Although shattered, most parts, relatively speaking, were in the right places, with the wings sticking out from the fuselage in the normal place and not lying somewhere else.

The aircraft apparently belly flopped into a gully, hitting the odd tree and slithering up the higher far side. The fuselage snapped in at least two places, with one break right behind the flight deck, so that the nose, with the flight crew inside, flipped over the brow to land near a house. Lack of fuel meant there was no fire, but the great g-forces of the impact meant all 85 survivors were injured.

Of the 158 persons on board, 73 died, mostly due to head and upper-body injuries. Three doctors involved in the treatment of the injured wrote a paper analyzing the injuries, suggesting it might provide valuable lessons regarding better constraints for passengers. Cost-benefit considerations meant that not all suggestions would be implemented.

As regards passenger survival, this accident was somewhat atypical in that the aircraft had completely empty tanks and getting out before succumbing to the effects of smoke inhalation was not the key to survival.

Causes

As usual, a whole series of factors were responsible for the disaster:

1. Lack of assertiveness on the part of the first officer, perhaps explained by an inferiority complex when dealing with the, in his mind, "superior" American controllers. At one point the flight engineer had even remarked that the controller sounded angry, when this does not seem to be the case.

2. Hoping for the optimum scenario, though the controller at the outset might have done better to suggest a more probable hold time rather than saying "at least forty-five minutes."

3. The creeping up of events, in that they remained on hold for so long that the option of diverting to their alternate, Boston, was lost. This could be classed as indecision.

4. The first officer handling the radio communications did not even once use the word "emergency," though he was told specifically to do so by the captain.

5. Neither did he inform the tower that their attempt to land was in fact their one and only chance, in which case the controller using radar could have tried to talk them down until they could see the runway.

    Admittedly, they were expecting it to be a routine landing, but even so, by informing the controller it was their last chance would have meant he or she would have done their utmost to avoid ordering a go-around.

6. Finally, there was a fatal dose of bad luck in that just as they were coming down toward the runway, expecting everything to be finally all right, they had to raise the nose and add power to regain height lost due to the wind shear, and probably thereby failed to pick out the runway in the murk.

FAA Held Partly Responsible by Court

ATC was under great pressure, having to cope with so many aircraft holding in the difficult weather conditions, and having to order some to go around because of lack of separation.

Had this not been so, the controllers might have felt able to devote time to exploring what the first officer meant when he repeatedly told them—but different controllers—that the aircraft was running out of fuel, something that would have been true to a greater or lesser extent for many of the aircraft they were handling at the time.

However, the courts subsequently made the FAA, as the controllers' employer, liable for 40 percent of the $200 million awarded as compensation.

Unnecessary Fatalities—Frail Seat Attachments

The broken off parts of the fuselage were mostly intact; the deceleration had not been too brutal and there was no fuel to produce a fire.

More people should therefore have survived.

That they did not was because the frail seat attachments on the cabin floor had hardly been improved since the sixties, and passengers were hurtled forward in their seats with them pilling up on each other.

Some of those weak seats had become contorted with the passengers strapped in them suffering hip and spinal fractures.

The passengers had not been warned of the impending impact and the need to assume the brace position which might have saved some additional people despite the flimsy seats and fixations.

BA 777 from Beijing Loses Thrust on Late Final (Heathrow, 2008)

Captain who saved them by reducing flap bad-mouthed

> It took a considerable time for the investigators to demonstrate how and why the interruption of the fuel supply to the engines occurred.
>
> British Airways Flight 38, January 17, 2008

A fter a long flight from Beijing, which only differed from many others in that the aircraft flew through some exceptionally cold air early on, the British Airways Boeing 777 was coming in quite normally to land at London's Heathrow's Runway 27L. As is usual after what is virtually a long, steady glide under the new arrangement to save fuel, a little extra thrust was required at the last minute to prevent the aircraft losing too much airspeed and sinking below the glide path.

To the pilots' dismay, this was not forthcoming, and it looked as if the aircraft was destined to touch down just before reaching the airport.

The first officer was flying the aircraft at the time, and although normally the captain takes over in a crisis, the captain let him continue—an apparently sensible decision, as the first officer had the feel of the aircraft and there was so little time left. The captain reduced the amount of flap to 25 percent, thus reducing the drag and allowing the aircraft to fly farther. The aircraft staggered over the perimeter fence and came down heavily on the grass just beyond, some thousand feet short of the paved runway.

The right main landing gear broke off, while the force of the impact forced the landing gear on the left into the wing. The first officer managed to keep the aircraft in a straight line and thus prevent it from cartwheeling. After skidding across the grass, it ended up just at the beginning of the runway paving.

Despite an escape of fuel due to the pilots' failure to switch off the fuel supply to the engines correctly, there was no fire and there were no fatalities. The 136 passengers and 16 crew members evacuated the aircraft via the chutes, with one passenger suffering a broken leg. The airline and no doubt its insurers soon deemed the aircraft not worth repairing and classed it as a write-off.

Initially, the media reported many passengers considered it a nonevent, with some only thinking it had been a hard landing. Their main gripe seemed to be their insensitive treatment on reaching the terminal. Yet some days later, with the arrival of lawyers on the scene, some were talking of the great distress they had suffered as justification for suing the airline.

This in turn led to the CEO of BA personally contacting passengers to head off legal action by showing personal concern.

In this context, one might mention that some at BA think there are business- and first-class passengers who regard the airline as a soft touch in that they greatly exaggerate their suffering when things go wrong in order to obtain free flights and/or upgrades. Passengers in economy are not treated so benignly by the airline.

That said, there were injuries and one Australian man sitting in seat 30K had his leg crushed when a 12-inch cylindrical beam of the front wheel assembly pierced the skin of the fuselage. Luckily, he was not in the brace position with his head near his knees.

In their preliminary report the UK's Air Accident Investigation Board (AAIB) concluded that ice in the fuel was the probable cause and recommended modifications to the fuel supply system on 777s fitted with Rolls-Royce engines. While it was not possible at that time to find cast-iron proof that ice in the fuel was the cause, concern increased, as there had been another case where an engine of a 777 flying in cold conditions had temporarily lost power.

The NTSB, the US equivalent of the AAIB, was far more forceful in its recommendations, announced simultaneously with those issued by the AAIB, which the UK investigators regarded as bad form. The NTSB maintained that interim precautionary measures, such as coming down to warmer air rather than staying high up, could expose aircraft to greater risk than usual.

Cause Finally Proven

The UK investigators looked at every conceivable reason for the engines to not respond but failed to find anything wrong with the computers or the programming. Indeed, the valves supplying fuel to the engines had opened fully in response to the demand for more thrust.

The quality of the fuel itself was checked and found to be above average. It was from South Korea and had been shipped to a Chinese port and sent directly by pipeline to Beijing Airport. Investigators found some matter in the fuel tanks, no doubt left there at the time of manufacture.

The investigators concluded that ice must have been the cause, but despite numerous attempts over many months, they were unable to replicate a situation where ice formed on the inside of the fuel pipes and broke off to block the fuel/lubricating oil heat exchanger.

They compared the flight in question with thousands of other flights and found that although the weather over Russia had been exceptionally cold, the pilots had constantly checked that the temperature of the fuel never fell to the level where it would become waxy. There was only one case where a Rolls-Royce engine on a 777 had behaved similarly. However, that had happened to a Delta aircraft at cruising height and only involved a single engine and had resolved itself when the pilot throttled back before reapplying power, something the BA pilots obviously could not have done in their predicament.

Finally, investigators noted again that the aircraft had flown for hours so precisely on autothrottle that there had never been a demand for a surge in power. The simple conclusion was that this allowed ice to build up inside the fuel pipes and remain there until the sudden demand for power prior to landing. They noted that this had been true in the case of the Delta 777 too.

Replicating the situation in tests, they found ice built up on the inside of the pipes, and when a sudden demand for high power was invoked, the ice broke off in such quantities that the heat exchanger was blocked. The cause had been proven conclusively, much to the relief of the many users of the Boeing 777.

The problem only pertained to 777s fitted with Rolls-Royce engines, because the tubes in their heat exchangers carrying the fuel through the hot oil protruded a few millimeters from the part carrying the oil and could not melt large quantities of ice deposited on them when cold fuel was flowing. Incidentally, the pilot of the Delta 777 unblocked the exchanger by throttling back and giving the ice time to melt.

The temporary solution was to power up the engines from time to time to prevent the buildup of ice inside the pipes. The long-term solution was to redesign the heat exchanger.

Sour Aftertaste

An unwarranted whispering campaign largely among cabin crew at the airline that Captain Burkill had frozen at the controls finally led to him resigning in disgust, only for him to find no other serious airline would employ him.

Even though Captain Burkill was blameless, any pilot involved in a serious incident can have difficulty finding employment elsewhere, and in his case the rumors did not help. Falling on relatively hard times, he wrote a well-received book, *Thirty Seconds to Impact*, in conjunction with his wife about the incident and its aftermath. Finally, British Airways reinstated him.

Poisoned Chalice

Captain Burkill makes a very interesting point about how accolades can be a poisoned chalice and cites a case at BA during the writing of the book where BA pilots had very probably saved the lives of all on board through fantastic airmanship. They had refused medals, preferring to stay anonymous, having seen for themselves how such recognition can lead to problems.

Chapter 3
RUNWAY OVERRUNS

"Safest Airline's" 100 mph Overrun (Bangkok, 1999)
747 aquaplaned after captain canceled go-around

> Australia's Qantas airline mostly flies long-haul routes to the world's major airports, where there is relatively little risk. With good pilots and an absence of bad luck, it could boast of never having suffered a hull loss (in the jet age).
>
> The airline came close to blotting its copybook in stormy weather in Bangkok, and indeed only avoided doing so by carrying out the most expensive repairs ever made to a civilian aircraft.
>
> Qantas Flight 001, September 23, 1999

Looking out from the twenty-eighth-floor balcony of a tower apartment on the bank of Bangkok's Chao Phraya River, the author watched torrential rain of an intensity he had never witnessed. He wondered how pilots of incoming aircraft could cope with it. As if in answer to that question, the next day's *Bangkok Post* had a few lines saying a Qantas 747 had been involved in some trouble at the airport, with no injuries. The incident was termed a mere mishap. However, when more details became available, perhaps through disaffected Qantas staff, the "mishap" became headline news in Thailand.

Apparently, the jumbo was still traveling at 100 miles an hour (160 kilometers an hour) when it ran onto the grass at the end of the paved runway overrun area after coming in to land. The *Bangkok Post* was later to comment, "It was a miracle a fire leading to many deaths had not occurred," adding that the landing had also been a "fiasco" in that, as explained later, some systems on the aircraft "assumed" it was about to take off, which for a moment it was.

The Thai authorities were miffed to discover Qantas staff had removed the quick access data recorder but finally asked the then highly respected Australian Transport Safety Bureau (ATSB) to investigate the incident. After all, in the absence of significant injuries, and with damage limited to Australian property, the Thais preferred to take a backseat.

How the Events Unfolded

Qantas 1, a Boeing 747 flight from Sydney to London with an intermediate stop at Bangkok, first nosed into the exceptionally heavy rain at a height of 200 feet, and with just 930 yards (850 meters) to go before crossing the threshold of the slightly shorter of Bangkok Airport's two parallel runways. The aircrew, consisting of the captain, first officer, who was the pilot piloting the aircraft (PF), and second officer, were aware they would encounter difficult conditions, since the storms over the airport had long been visible on their weather radar. Now, at late final, the usually crisp white runway lights were only visible to the PF for brief moments after each pass of the windscreen wiper blades.

Another Qantas aircraft with call sign "Qantas 15," had been about three minutes ahead of them in the landing sequence but had decided to go around because of poor visibility. The crew of Qantas 1 were still on the approach control frequency and were not aware of this. Therefore, when they moved to the tower frequency and were informed that a Thai Airbus had landed ahead of them and "braking was good," they thought the interval was the usual three minutes, when in fact it had become six. This is a long time in a tropical storm. Had the tower told them their colleagues just ahead had abandoned their landing, their mind-set might well have been different.

As Qantas 1 descended in the downpour to 140 feet, the captain became concerned that while the aircraft had speeded up it had not descended sufficiently fast and said to the first officer:

You are getting high now!

Shortly afterward came the automatic voice warning that they were at a hundred feet.

The captain said:

You happy?

The first officer replied:

Ah, yes.

According to the ATSB report, the first officer later stated that he felt he was getting near his personal limits by this time but was happy to continue with the approach, as the captain appeared to be happy. He maintained that he had the feel of the aircraft, and it made more sense for him to continue rather than hand over control at that point. The second officer also reported that he was comfortable with continuing the approach at that stage. (The first officer had decided to carry out the approach manually rather than use the autopilot to "keep his hand in.")

On crossing the runway threshold, they were thirty-two feet *above* the ideal height, almost fifteen knots *above* the target speed, and nineteen knots above the reference speed, V_{REF}. These excesses were individually just within company limits. At the same time, the distorting effect of the rivulets of water on the windscreen would certainly have made it difficult for the first officer to judge distances correctly.

The fifty-foot-altitude warning sounded, and the nose went up slightly, resulting in the aircraft prematurely beginning its flare[1] and prompting the captain to say:

> *Get it down! Get it down! Come on, you're starting your flare.*

Acknowledging this, the first officer began to retard the engine thrust levers in preparation for touchdown. The rate of descent, which had already dropped to approximately five feet a second, slowed even further due to the flare.

The first officer later reported that although the reduced visibility made it difficult to judge the landing flare, they were already in it and thought it best to pursue it and allow the aircraft to settle onto the runway. He believed that they had more than enough runway remaining for them to stop.

The thirty-foot warning marking the height they would normally have begun their flare sounded, with the longer-than-usual interval between the fifty-feet and thirty-feet calls indicating a slower-than-normal descent.

The captain, no doubt getting concerned about the delayed touchdown, increased the autobrake setting to "4" without advising the other crew members, as it did not materially affect the touchdown.

With only ten feet left before the dangling main wheels would first touch the runway, the captain ordered a go-around. He felt the aircraft was "floating," and he could not see the far end of the runway. In addition, he was not happy with the speed, which again was within company limits, but at the upper limit of what he personally was prepared to accept.

Instead of using the takeoff/go-around (TOGA) switch, which would have reconfigured the aircraft automatically for takeoff, the first officer initiated the go-around by pushing the engine thrust levers forward. This is quite common practice, as the automatic TOGA go-around controlled by the aircraft's computers can be a little alarming to passengers, since it is abrupt and indelicate, on the assumption that it may be an emergency. Anyway, the first officer reacted very quickly, so it did not make much difference, other than that a manual go-around is easier to cancel.

With the engines needing some eight to spool up from idle, the aircraft's main wheels would inevitably brush the runway before the aircraft could regain enough speed for positive lift.

Just then, when it seemed they were quite rightly going to forgo the landing in the name of safety, a letup in the rain allowed the captain to see right to the far end of the runway. Reassured, he decided to cancel the go-around.

Instead of announcing his intention, he put his hand over the first officer's, left hand resting on the throttles, to push them back. For a moment, the first officer was unsure who was flying the aircraft. Worse, one lever slipped from his grasp and remained where it was.

The 747's systems interpreted the fact that one lever was forward as an intention to take off and disarmed both the automatic braking and automatic deployment of the spoilers. (Spoilers are flat panels hinged at the front set on top of the wings that flick up to "spoil" the flow of air over the wing. This not only produces an air braking effect but also pushes the aircraft down, improving the grip of the tires on the runway.)

Having to pull the recalcitrant lever back to join the others in the idle position possibly made the first officer forget to apply reverse thrust.

Braking manually as hard as they could, the two pilots at the controls were shocked to find the usually exceptionally effective carbon brakes were hardly slowing the aircraft at all. This was particularly troubling, as having landed so far down the runway in the first place, and furthermore, having for a moment one engine thrusting them forward with no spoilers and no wheel brakes, meant even more of the remaining runway had been used up.

With the tires aquaplaning on the layer of water on what little runway remained, they ran onto the short overrun area and then onto the grass at an incredible 100 mph.

Fortunately, the heavy rain that had initially been their undoing ultimately proved their salvation, for the rain-sodden ground allowed the huge wheels to sink deeply into it, with the result that the aircraft finally came to rest some 240 yards (220 meters) farther on, without encountering any serious obstacle on the way.

The rain and wet ground may indeed have saved them a second time by quickly dousing any nascent fires. With the aircraft having come to a stop, the captain immediately reviewed the situation, made more difficult by the fact that wires for communicating with the cabin crew, as well as those for the PA (public address) system, had been severed, as they passed close to the crushed nose-wheel section. He could only get information piecemeal by messenger.

Only after waiting some twenty minutes and after the arrival of rescue vehicles did he order the evacuation.

The ATSB board of inquiry thought this delay in evacuation had been unwise, as the captain could not have been sure a fire would not break out. In addition, the batteries supplying power for the emergency lighting system were on the verge of giving out, as the designers did not anticipate emergency evacuations taking so long. If there had subsequently been a fire, an evacuation without even emergency lighting would have been a nightmare.

In the event, waiting for transport avoided injuries and the danger that the captain later mentioned of passengers being struck by aircraft when tempted to "walk over the adjacent busy runway towards the brightly lit terminal."

On board, there had been 3 aircrew, 16 cabin crew, and 391 passengers. None sustained significant physical injury.

Despite the soft ground, the aircraft itself sustained a considerable amount of damage and stress, as evidenced by the $75 million initial estimate for the cost of repairs.

Verdict—Not What You Might Expect

From the above account, one might immediately assume that the flight crew was responsible for the near disaster, and even culpable. Instead, the ATSB, relying very much on Professor Reason's Swiss cheese accident model—according to which accidents happen where all the holes (mistakes and faults) in the cheese line up—concluded that Qantas had not properly prepared its Boeing 747-400 pilots for landing on "contaminated" (in other words, water covered or icy runways).

Also, partly to reduce costs, had introduced a new, "less conservative" (more risky) standard landing procedure without proper consideration.

The ATSB report noted, "With the introduction of the more powerful carbon brakes, Qantas had changed their standard landing procedure to Flaps 25 idle reverse thrust rather than the previous more conservative Flaps 30 full reverse Thrust."

Flaps are movable extensions to the leading edge and trailing edge of the wings that configure the wing to give more lift, especially at low speed, when taking off or landing.

"Reverse thrust" simply means that cowlings on the engines move so that the thrust from the engine pushes the plane backward rather than forward. Before the introduction of the better-performing carbon brakes, passengers would almost invariably hear this engine roar just after landing. Incidentally, setting "Idle reverse" does little to slow the aircraft but means the transition to full reverse can be accomplished quickly.

Qantas made this change in landing procedure for financial and, to some extent, noise abatement reasons. It could save money because carbon brakes wear less if applied continuously rather than intermittently. In addition, with a flap angle of 25 degrees, there is less wear on the flap mechanism. Not using full reverse thrust would also reduce maintenance costs for the thrust reverser mechanism. However, extra wear on the tires would negate some of these gains.

Comparison in the ATSB report with five other major airlines flying routes in Asia and worldwide—unnamed due to reasons of commercial confidentiality—showed the others to be more conservative:

1. Many stressed the need to be warier of storms and the need to use Flaps 30/full reverse thrust in heavy rain situations.

2. The other airlines had more experience than Qantas of flying into difficult airports.

Some Qantas pilots believed the more conservative Flaps 30 also made it easier to land precisely at the desired point—Qantas 1 landed well beyond the ideal touchdown point.

The crew of Qantas 1 did not even discuss the Flaps 30/full reverse option, even though their weather radar had revealed the storms over the airport when they were far away, with plenty of time.

The ATSB report said this was probably because, with the introduction of the new standard, landings were hardly ever made with Flaps 30, and they were unlikely to try something with which they were unfamiliar.

According to reference data supplied by Boeing, the aircraft *could not have stopped in time* on the contaminated runway using the standard Qantas Flaps 25 idle-reverse landing procedure. This remained true even if it had landed at the ideal touchdown point 400 yards (366 meters) from the threshold. However, it *could* have stopped if they had used full reverse thrust in addition and everything else had been ideal—that is to say, no canceled go-around and so on.

The whole incident could have been avoided had the captain not dismissed the first officer's earlier suggestion that they hold off to the south until the weather improved, saying it was only a shower. Their aircraft was not the only one trying to come in, so it was just a matter of opinion, bearing in mind that conditions can suddenly change in that part of the world.

The ATSB report cited the following adverse factors in the reverse order of their occurrence. The author's comments are in parentheses.

1. Reverse thrust
    Had they not in the turmoil forgotten to engage reverse thrust, even in the idling mode, as specified

in their standard landing instructions, there would have been a slight deceleration effect rather than the slight acceleration produced by idle forward. Many Qantas pilots said they occasionally forgot to engage reverse thrust when something distracted them. Normally, this would not have serious implications and therefore would not be uppermost in their minds. Of course, full reverse rather than idle reverse thrust would have been better.

2. Nonverbal cancellation of the go-around
    The captain, perhaps because it was a habit developed in the course of his frequent work training pilots, cancelled the go-around merely by putting his hand over that of the first officer to pull back the engine thrust levers. It was unlucky one lever remained forward with the consequences already mentioned, and as said, the first officer for a moment wondered who was flying the aircraft. Theoretically, this direct action by the captain would have averted the delay between his issuing the command to cancel the go-around and its execution.

3. Cancellation of go-around
    Pilots generally do not consider canceling a go-around to be good practice, as it can lead to confusion and other problems, as was indeed the case here.
    However, put yourself in the captain's place. There he was—so he thought—finally safely on the ground after a difficult landing.

In the atrocious weather conditions, a second landing might be even trickier, with not much reserve of fuel for a third attempt. Moreover, both he and the first officer were convinced there was more than enough runway to stop, which there would have been had it not been for the standing water on the runway. Ordering and subsequently canceling the go-around meant more runway was used up due to the engines beginning to power up, not to mention one engine continuing to pull because of the "lost" thrust lever, which in turn made the aircraft "think" it was taking off, which prevented immediate deployment of the spoilers and application of the brakes on touchdown.

4. Landing too far down the runway
    The first officer came in somewhat fast and too high and initiated the flare early, consequently touching down far along the runway. He attributed this partly to the heavy rain. (One point not stressed by the investigators was that the depth of the water at the beginning of the runway where aircraft normally land—and where the Airbus six minutes ahead found braking had been "good"—was doubtless less deep than at the other end, because landing aircraft would have splashed it away. If he had touched down earlier, braking might have been sufficient to reduce the speed enough to prevent aquaplaning on reaching that presumably deeper water.)

5. No prior decision to use safer Flaps 30 with full reverse thrust

    The crew's experience of trouble-free landings in heavy rain in places such as Bangkok and Singapore may have made it overlook the possible severity of some patches of rain in Thailand.

6. Qantas had abandoned use of windscreen water repellent

    Qantas had abandoned the use of water repellent on Boeing 747s, deactivating the systems several years before for financial reasons and ostensibly to protect the environment—water repellents consist of fluorocarbons that cause depletion of the ozone layer. (It is perhaps true, as some Qantas pilots maintain that water repellents do not in general make much difference.

    [The author's personal experience of driving in Thailand showed that in torrential downpours they make an incredible difference to visibility through the windscreen, even well after the wiper blades have passed. Thus, merely the use of water repellent could have greatly changed the scenario: the first officer might not have landed so far down the runway, and the captain might have been able to see the far end of the runway early on and not have ordered the go-around in the first place.]

7. Second officer's wife

    The ATSB report discounts the presence of the second officer's wife in the cockpit as an adverse factor in the incident, but could concern for his spouse have led to a moment's inattention, causing the second officer to miss noting the first officer had not applied idle reverse?

8. Autopilot not used

The first officer flew the aircraft manually to get more hands-on practice. (Furthermore, the diffractive effect of the layer of water on the windscreen would have made it difficult for the first officer to judge the distance correctly. The aircraft would surely have come in at the slower correct speed and touched down near the optimum point on the runway had the first officer flying the aircraft [PF] opted to use the automatic pilot. This would have given an extra 636 meters, not to mention the already stated fact that the beginning of the runway might well have had less water on it, partly because aircraft landing there would have dispersed it. Had it not been for the standing water, his landing would have been just about acceptable.)

Conclusion

Qantas, in the inquiry's view, seemed to have erred in not training pilots suitably for coping with contaminated runways. Though Boeing said the aircraft could not have stopped in time with the given configuration even had everything, apart from the aquaplaning, been perfect, in the author's opinion the overrun would only have been slight, and most airports have some spare space at the end of their runways for such eventualities.

It was the combination of so many other negatives that made this a potential disaster, which would have been the case had the soggy ground not slowed the aircraft. Had there been solid obstacles earlier in the path of the aircraft as it hurtled off the runway, any one of these factors could have meant the difference between life and death for hundreds of people.

In response, Qantas introduced changes in its training and management to avoid such an incident happening again. As usual, other airlines learned from this mishap at no cost to themselves.

In May 2000, after being repaired in China, that same aircraft had to turn back on a flight out of Hong Kong because of generator problems. According to the *Sydney Morning Herald*, a Qantas engineer, who did not wish to be named, told it that he and his colleagues had predicted such electrical problems "because of the quality of workmanship in China." One should note, however, that the *Sydney Morning Herald* said Qantas's chief executive, James Strong, denied that Qantas had had the aircraft repaired rather than scrapped, just so Qantas could maintain its claim that it had never had a hull loss. According to Mr. Strong, the $100 million cost of the repairs only represented 40 percent of the cost of the aircraft. However, there is no mention in this of the scrap value, as parts could surely have been reused.

In addition, there were probably considerable additional costs in terms of the Qantas management time required to oversee the repair project in China. People who have flown in the repaired aircraft have noted how the front looks newer than the back.

Personnel Changes at Qantas

Very often airlines and organizations wait quite some time before officially announcing personnel changes after an accident. To bolster its position, the airline will initially express full confidence in those involved, only to let them go later, as was the case for the Singapore Airlines pilots involved in the takeoff from the disused runway at Taipei, where two of the three were later dismissed. Did the same apply at Qantas after the incident just described?

One wonders, because on May 30, 2003, the *Australian* featured the startling headline "Qantas Safety Tsar's Reign Ends." According to the article, Ken Lewis (the "tsar" in question) had "left the job after twenty-three years as head of safety and almost four decades at the airline." It added that he would continue to advise senior management until leaving the airline.

The paper emphasized that he was highly respected throughout the industry, "having qualified as a meteorologist, worked as a flight attendant, as a ground simulator instructor and navigation instructor, and is a qualified air safety instructor." He had held positions on international safety bodies and was at the time president of the Australian Society of Air Safety Investigators.

Though he was certainly a good man—incidentally, more problems seem to have occurred since his replacement—one wonders whether his qualifications would have given him the mind-set and clout to influence senior Qantas management (including the bean counters) in the manner the investigators thought necessary in this particular case.

The article in the *Australian* also mentioned that the airline was replacing its chief pilot and returning him to line flying. Possibly, the moves were prompted by the fact that the airline was under investigation regarding another incident, in which a 737 landing in rainy conditions veered off the runway for a while at Darwin after a heavy touchdown just beyond the normal runway threshold. Again, no one was injured, but there was some damage to the tires and flaps.

However, on January 13, 2008, the *Sydney Morning Herald*, in an article about the slide in Qantas's share value and Merrill Lynch's sell recommendation, said the carrier a week previously had suffered "arguably the biggest dent to its once-enviable safety reputation in decades" after one of its Boeing 747s lost electrical power on approach to Bangkok. It was referring to a Boeing 747-400 London-to-Bangkok flight that lost electrical power from all four engine-driven electrical generators fifteen minutes out of Bangkok and had to rely on backup power to land there.

Battery power would only have lasted for about an hour, and had the aircraft been a long way from an airport and in bad weather, the situation could have been precarious. Unlike many twin-engine aircraft, the four-engine 747 is not fitted with a RAT, a ram air turbine, to generate emergency electric power while gliding.

Investigators found the loss of electrical power had been caused by water entering the electrical equipment bay through cracks in the drip shield above it. Checks found similar cracks in the shields of other 747-400s in the Qantas fleet, and all were repaired. Whether there is any direct connection, but a court case was to proceed regarding a Qantas engineer with allegedly fake qualifications who had worked on that model of aircraft.

Airlines do go through periods where one problem after another crops up and often end up better as a result, and those mentioned were some time ago.

---

[1] The landing flare (usually performed at a height of about 30 feet) consists of raising the aircraft nose to produce (1) *extra lift* to break the descent and (2) *extra drag* to slow the aircraft so it subsequently sinks onto the runway. It is rather like a big bird landing, except that birds can lower their "flaps" and do a flare dramatically at the very last instant, which passenger aircraft cannot.

Air France A340 Overruns, Catches Fire in Gully (Toronto, 2005)
Passengers collecting hand baggage impede evacuation

> Even though on reaching the end of the runway the Air France A340 at Toronto was traveling twenty knots slower than Qantas's 747 at Bangkok, there was little clear ground beyond.
>
> That ground was not soft enough to have a significant braking effect, and in addition there was a gully lying ahead.
>
> Air France Flight 358, August 2, 2005

J ust as with the Qantas 747 at Bangkok, the Air France Airbus A340 from Paris was being flown manually as it came in to land in a storm at Toronto's Lester B. Pearson International Airport. This meant that when the throttles were pushed forward to compensate for a sudden switch to a tail component to the wind, they stayed forward longer than would have been the case under autothrottle. This in turn contributed to the aircraft passing over the runway threshold at seventy to eighty feet, some forty meters higher than usual.

The rain and poor visibility then made it difficult to bring the aircraft down quickly, and as a result it touched down more than two-fifths of the way down the 9,000-foot (2,743-meter) runway at 143 knots (274 km/h) IAS (indicated airspeed), with only 5,250 feet (1,600 meters) of runway left.

The spoilers duly deployed after three seconds and maximum manual breaking was applied.

Yet idle reverse thrust was only selected 12.8 seconds after touchdown (at IAS 118 km/h, with only 670 meters of runway remaining), and full reverse only after 16.4 seconds with even less runway left.

These delays can be attributed to the pilot flying (PF) concentrating on keeping the aircraft on the runway in the relatively strong crosswind, and the fact that attention was not drawn to the failure to apply reverse thrust, as the pilot not flying (PNF) was not making the customary announcements confirming deployment of the spoilers and thrust reversers.

Unable to stop in time, the aircraft departed the runway at eighty-six knots corrected ground speed, passing over a grassy area and then a road before ending up in a minor ravine. Most of the damage to the aircraft occurred in the ravine.

With fire breaking out, an emergency evacuation was ordered. Ignoring instructions from the cabin crew not to do so, almost half the passengers retrieved their carry-on baggage. One man even blocked an aisle as he busied himself rearranging items in his case. Ignoring angry comments from passengers standing behind him and orders from the flight attendant to leave his baggage and go to the emergency exit, he persisted, obliging the attendant to redirect passengers through the middle bank of seats to the other side of the aircraft to gain access to the only available emergency exit in the aft cabin.

Because there was fire on one side blocking two slides and another was punctured by debris, some people were injured in the course of jumping from a considerable height.

Moments after the last person exited the aircraft it was engulfed in flames, so it was a close-run thing, and the bringing of luggage almost resulted in fatalities.

Of the 309 people on board, 12 (2 crew and 10 passengers) suffered serious injuries, nine of which were incurred at the time of impact, and three during the evacuation. The two members of the cabin crew who were seriously injured were hurt at the time of impact but were still able to perform their duties. Passengers with serious impact injuries were nevertheless able to walk.

At the time, the airport was on red alert because of rain and lightning, and some have argued that the control tower should not have permitted the landing, with others saying the decision was up to the captain, who had enough fuel to divert.

Air France Culture and PR Spin

The freelance French aviation writer François Hénin cites this poor landing as an example of laxness at the airline, though some have suggested the delayed touchdown and too fast approach was due to a microburst producing a tail wind during the latter part of the approach. However, failure of the PNF to make the customary callouts confirming deployment of the spoilers and thrust reversers certainly did constitute laxness.

He also points out how the Air France PR department cleverly flooded the media with glowing accounts of the "truly remarkable job" the Air France cabin crew had done when their performance had merely been appropriate, thus diverting attention from what could have been a tragic disaster with the airline apparently at fault. The aircraft ended up a burnt-out wreck. It was the first significant accident involving an Airbus A340 in 14 years of operation.

Other Elements

The control tower in addition to clearing the aircraft to land on Runway 24L warned them the preceding aircraft had reported braking action to be poor. This should have readied the pilots to abort the landing in the event of their not being able to touch down close to the threshold.

As they came in too high, the captain said, "Put it down! Put it down!"

Deciding to do a go-around when finding one is touching down much too far down the runway is a balance of risks and a difficult decision with no time for hesitation. However, on top of coming down too late, the critical factor seems to have been the late deployment of full reverse thrust. Had it been initiated eighteen seconds earlier the aircraft might still have overrun but not necessarily have caught fire.

When questioned about this, the captain claimed the copilot flying tensed up because of the difficulty he was having controlling the aircraft in the wind on the slippery runway and was gripping the throttles so tightly that he (the captain not flying) could not set full reverse thrust.

This hardly makes   sense, as he or she normally would verbally confirm they had set full reverse thrust, or if not needed to do so.

Chapter 4
MIDAIR COLLISIONS
AND TCAS

Midair Collisions at Grand Canyon and New York City (1956, 1960)

Air traffic control in the US was then very primitive

These midair collisions were a wake-up call.

TWA Flight 2 and UA Flight 718, June 30, 1956
UA Flight 826 and TWA Flight 266, December 16, 1960

TWA Flight 2 Collides with UA Flight 718
at the Grand Canyon

On June 30, 1956, two aircraft took off at around nine o'clock in the morning from adjacent runways at Los Angeles International Airport. The first was Transworld Airlines Lockheed Super Constellation Flight 2 bound for Kansas City, with sixty-four passengers and six crew. The second, only three minutes later, was United Airlines Douglas DC-7 Flight 718 bound for Chicago, with fifty-three passengers and five crew.

The DC-7 was the first airliner able to fly almost one hundred passengers across the US from coast to coast nonstop. US Airways was justifiably proud of it, though it was soon to be superseded by the Boeing 707 and other jet airliners.

Its powerful engines were fault prone, and ultimately more DC-6s than DC-7s remained in long-term service.

Each aircraft climbed out of Los Angeles along a different controlled airway, with the one taken by the TWA Constellation taking it northeast to a waypoint at Daggett, roughly in line with its eventual route. That followed by the DC-7 took it southwest to one at Palm Springs, more off its eventual route. After they had adjusted course at these waypoints, it so happened that, due to the DC-7's 18 knot (20 mph) higher airspeed, the aircraft would cross paths simultaneously an hour after takeoff in an area just before the so-called "Painted Desert" line. This should not have presented a problem, with the Constellation flying at nineteen thousand feet and the DC-7 at twenty-one thousand feet.

The term Painted Desert line is somewhat confusing, as it suggests a line in the desert. In fact, it was the name given by air traffic control to a virtual line about two hundred miles long running north-northwest between the VOR radio beacons at Winslow, Arizona, and Bryce Canyon, Utah. Passing to the east of the Grand Canyon, it traversed an area of beautiful rock formations in striated colors that was called the "Painted Desert" (El Desierto Pintado) by an expedition under Francisco Vázquez de Coronado in 1540, hence the name.

In 1956, air traffic control in the US was very primitive and, in many areas, virtually nonexistent. After all, the country was enormous, and airliners were so few that apart from areas where they would be funneled (bunch up), there was plenty of room for them to avoid each other when flying under visual flight rules, following the principle of "see and be seen."

Furthermore, other than in the vicinity of large cities or the airport of departure or arrival, the controllers did not contact the aircraft directly but usually through the intermediary of the airline's dispatchers. In vast uncontrolled areas with no radar coverage, pilots would report to their companies when passing over the waypoints on their route.

At 9:21, the Constellation reported that it was approaching the Daggett waypoint and requested a change in cruising height from nineteen thousand to twenty-one thousand feet to try and avoid cumulonimbus clouds building up over the Grand Canyon area. The dispatcher contacted air traffic control at Los Angeles Center, who in turn contacted Salt Lake City control center, which covered the airspace TWA was about to enter.

The Los Angeles controller, aware the United Airlines DC-7 would be crossing paths with the Constellation at precisely that altitude, doubted it would be possible, and the Salt Lake City controller confirmed.

The Los Angeles controller contacted the airline to say the request for twenty-one thousand could not be approved, to which the TWA dispatcher replied, "Just a minute. I think he wants a thousand on top; yes, a thousand on top until he can get it."

Here the captain of the Constellation was exploiting a regulation that said that if flying under visual flight rules, where the pilots are responsible for looking out for each other's craft, they can request to fly one thousand feet above the clouds or overcast. On being assured TWA 2 would be at least one thousand feet above the clouds, the Los Angeles controller duly gave permission, and as a result the Constellation ended up cruising at precisely the altitude that had just been refused. However, unlike the DC-7, the Constellation was warned of the presence of the other in the vicinity. The Constellation even confirmed to the dispatcher that the United Flight 718 was at twenty-one thousand feet. That was not much help, as the DC- 7 would be overtaking from the side and behind.

Although "one thousand above" suggested the Constellation flying under visual flight rules would have been above all clouds, this was not true, for some clouds rose to twenty-five thousand feet, and the aircraft would have to skirt around them. The pilots of both aircraft would also have been positioning their aircraft to give their passengers some wonderful views of the scenery below, notably the Grand Canyon.

At approximately 9:58, United 718 made a position report to the CAA communications station at Needles stating that the flight was over Needles at twenty-one thousand feet and estimated that it would reach the Painted Desert line at 10:31. Surprisingly, only a minute later, at 9:59, TWA 2 reported to the TWA dispatcher at Las Vegas that it had passed Lake Mohave at the Arizona border at 9:55, was "a thousand feet on top," at twenty-one thousand feet, and would be reaching the Painted Desert line at 10:31.

No further communication was heard from the Constellation.

At 10:31 an unintelligible transmission was heard by aeronautical radio communicators at Salt Lake City and San Francisco, who had a contract with United to handle radio traffic. When it was played back later, they worked out that it must have been from the captain of the DC-7 saying they were about to crash: "Salt Lake, United 718 . . . uh . . . we're going in."

With no radar coverage, knowing where the aircraft were depended on receiving their reports over the radio as they passed waypoints, and sometimes pilots forgot to give them, which was the reason that the respective dispatchers were not overly concerned when there was no report at 10:31 of the aircraft passing over the Painted Desert line. However, when there were no reports at subsequent waypoints concern grew.

At 10:51, air traffic control at Salt Lake City, which covered the area where the two aircraft should be flying, received a call from United saying that the DC-7 was twenty minutes overdue at Painted Desert. Shortly afterwards they received a call from TWA saying the Constellation was also twenty minutes overdue at Painted Desert. Two aircraft "forgetting" to report was highly unlikely, and with everyone getting more worried, Salt Lake City tried to raise them every couple of minutes, while dispatchers tried various frequencies. After an hour of fruitless attempts to make contact, Salt Lake City telegraphed local authorities to see whether they had any information. There were no reports of anything untoward, and because the aircraft were not tracked by radar, looking for debris in that vast area would be like looking for a needle in a haystack.

Palen and Henry Hudgin, brothers who operated a small plane taking tourists on overflights of the Grand Canyon, heard about the search and remembered seeing smoke earlier in the day. They went back to look that evening and found the wreckage of an aircraft high up on an escarpment on the side of the canyon. The following morning, they saw the wreckage of another aircraft on the bed of the canyon, clearly identifiable as the Constellation due to its unique triple empennage.

Though marveled at by tourists—usually from above— the Grand Canyon is inhospitable, dangerous, and inaccessible. The first task was to get people in to see if there were any survivors, however unlikely that might be. Reaching the debris of the DC-7 high up on the side of the canyon proved especially difficult, and United Airlines brought in a team of Swiss mountaineers, who happened to be climbing not too far away. However, they found no survivors. In fact, there were hardly any identifiable bodies at either site, and much of the wreckage had fused to the rocks in the fires.

The total death toll was 128.

Investigation

At the time the Civil Aeronautics Board (CAB) was responsible for air accident investigations, but it was in its infancy and lacked the tools, such as flight data and cockpit voice recorders, that it has today. There were no witnesses either.

It was immediately obvious from the fact that the empennage of the Constellation was some distance from the rest of the wreckage that it had come off in flight. Likewise, the left wing outside panel of the DC-7 had separated in flight.

From red paint markings from the Constellation on the DC-7, and those from the DC-7 on the Constellation, it was possible to work out that the DC-7 had struck the Constellation coming downward and moving right to left, shearing off the tail empennage.

The details other than the direction and angle are not so important. They show that the faster DC-7 was coming from above and slightly behind, meaning the Constellation would not have been able to see it.

The person in charge of the difficult investigation carried out experiments to determine how difficult it would be for the pilots of the DC-7 to see the Constellation and concluded that as it would be in the peripheral vision, it might not be obvious if not moving from side to side.

There were, of course, other explanations.

1. The two aircraft could have been on either side of a cloud and come upon each other with little time to react;

2. The pilots might have been distracted by having to monitor their engines;

3. Or looking down to ensure their passengers got the best view of the Grand Canyon.

Air traffic control seemed to be a system with rules that everyone had followed, or in the case of the captain of the Constellation, exploited, with no one responsible other than the pilots over vast areas. Even as the two aircraft climbed out of Los Angeles in a controlled airway under instrument flight rules, they were asked to switch to visual flight rules, making avoiding other aircraft their responsibility.

People wonder why the Constellation was warned of the presence of the DC-7 and not the latter of that of the Constellation. Apparently, this was because it was not controlled airspace and not the controllers' business, and other aircraft could have been present as well, anyway. When the controller was asked about this, he said his statement about the presence of the DC-7 had not in fact been an "advisory" but merely an explanation as to why he had not been able to grant the request for a change in altitude to twenty-one thousand feet!

As a result of this crash and numerous similar but less deadly ones that had occurred in previous years, the Federal Aviation Agency was created in 1958. Its name was changed to the Federal Aviation Administration (FAA) in 1967, and responsibility for investigating air crashes was transferred from the CAB to the newly established NTSB.

Air traffic control was subsequently greatly improved, and the whole country was eventually covered with sophisticated radar able to warn controllers of a risk of collision.

Technology has made a great difference, notably the introduction of TACAS (traffic [alert and] collision avoidance system, now referred to as TCAS), which alerts pilots to the presence of other aircraft in their vicinity, and if a collision looks imminent even orders one to go up and the other down so they do not turn into each other, as people often do when coming suddenly toward each other in the street.

UA Flight 826 Collides with TWA Flight 266 at New York City

This midair collision at New York City was very different from the one at the Grand Canyon in that both aircraft were under direct air traffic control and flying under instrument flight rules. It was the first time information from an airliner's flight data recorder featured significantly in an air crash investigation.

The first aircraft involved was a United Airlines DC-8 four-engine jetliner, with seventy-seven passengers and a crew of seven, that had departed Chicago O'Hare Airport and was bound for New York's Idlewild Airport, now called JFK.

The second aircraft, which had thirty-nine passengers and five crew, was a slower Trans World Airlines piston-engine Lockheed Super Constellation that had come from Dayton, with a stopover at Port Columbus, and was bound for New York's LaGuardia Airport.

Though air traffic control was not informed, the pilot of the DC-8 had told United Airlines that one of its VOR receivers was not working.

The aircraft approached New York at the same time as the DC-8, at 10:25, allowed to take a shortcut to a point called Preston, where it was to hold, circling at five thousand feet, and at no more than 210 knots. Preston was not a beacon but the point where radials from beacons and an airway intersected.

For one reason or another—United Airlines later claimed one of those beacons was not working properly—the DC-8 overshot Preston, and at a higher speed than it should have been traveling, going eleven miles beyond it.

The TWA Constellation coming in to land at Idlewild was allowed to turn right slightly early to intersect the line leading to the runway, at which point it would turn left to line up with it. Though the TWA pilots had been warned of jet traffic to the right, no one imagined it would be where it was.

The engine of the DC-10 struck the fuselage of the Constellation, which broke up. Though parts were found far away, most fell onto the relatively open ground of Miller Army Airfield below. All forty-four people on board died, but no one on the ground was killed.

Having lost an engine and a great part of a wing, the DC-8 flew on, with some observers believing the pilots were trying to land, though the aircraft was doubtless uncontrollable.

It crashed on the Park Slope section of Brooklyn, setting fire to houses and buildings, immediately killing all but one of the 128 occupants but, considering it is such a densely populated area, luckily only six people on the ground.

Pictures of the carnage in the streets were shown all around the world, with the story given extra legs by the fact that an eleven-year-old boy was miraculously thrown from the fuselage onto a bank of snow, which broke his fall.

Residents rolled him in the snow to cool him and extinguish his smoldering clothes and found he could talk. He was a wonderful boy in all respects. A miracle amidst disaster. Sadly, he died of pneumonia the following day because his lungs had been seared by burning jet fuel.

Aftermath

A new regulation was brought in that required pilots operating under instrument flight rules to report all malfunctions of navigation or communication equipment.

A 250-knot speed limit near airports was also implemented.

Furthermore, the accident led to the installation of DME (distance measuring equipment) in aircraft showing the distance from radio beacons, and the FAA was prompted to modernize the air traffic control system through a task force reporting to President Kennedy.

PSA 182 727 Collides with Cessna (San Diego, 1978)

Pilot error, but contributing factors

> The improvements in air traffic control following the two midair collisions just described meant there was never another collision between airliners in the US.
>
> However, about twenty years later there was one between a Boeing 727 trijet and a general aviation Cessna piloted by a young man wearing a hood for instrument flying training.
>
> Pacific Southwest Airlines Flight 182 and Cessna, September 25, 1978

The Pacific Southwest Airlines 727 twinjet was approaching San Diego Airport, which unlike most major airports in the United States is nestled close to the city, making it more difficult to see small aircraft against a background of buildings. Being so confined, it is a challenging airport for pilots besides being the busiest single-runway airport in the States.

It was a bright, sunny day with visibility ten miles. On board the aircraft were 7 crew and 128 passengers, including 29 of the airline's employees. The pilot flying was First Officer Robert Fox, thirty-eight, and in the left-hand seat was Captain James McFeron, forty-two. With them was the obligatory flight engineer, and in the jump seat, and a source of distraction, was an off-duty PSA captain.

At 8:59, ATC alerted them to the presence nearby of a Cessna 172 Skyhawk, a very small GA aircraft that had taken off from Montgomery Field executive airport six miles from downtown San Diego and was legally operating under visual flight rules (VFR). This meant that they had not had to file a flight plan and only had to verbally signal their intentions to the controllers who could give them orders.

However, the pilot flying the Cessna was being trained to fly under instrument flight rules (IFR) and to make it realistic was wearing a hood restricting his vision to his instruments and controls. An instructor able to see outside was with him.

Though being piloted under IFR simulation, the Cessna was to the outside world performing a missed approach under visual meteorological conditions from San Diego's runway and climbing away to the east, and in contact with San Diego Approach Control. The Cessna without informing the controllers made a change in heading that bought it ahead of the faster airliner but below. The PSA 727 was descending.

Meanwhile the atmosphere in the cockpit of the PSA 727 had been very relaxed, with laughter and the off-duty captain telling an anecdote. They confirmed to ATC that they had seen the Cessna but not that they had subsequently lost sight of it. Nowadays, the sterile cockpit rule applied under ten thousand feet would have precluded this type of banter.

Just before they came down onto the Cessna:

09:01:11 The first officer said:

Are we clear of that Cessna?

09:01:13 Flight engineer:

Supposed to be.

09:01:14 Captain:

I guess.

[Laughter and unclear.]

09:01:20 Off-duty captain:

I hope.

09:01:21 Captain:

Oh yeah, before we turned downwind, I saw him at about one o'clock. Probably behind us now.

09:01:47

[Sound of impact.]

The impact with the Cessna severely damaged the 727's right wing, severed hydraulic lines, and made the aircraft uncontrollable. It pitched down to the right, with the fuel inside the wing catching fire.

As a last gesture, one and half seconds before the three-hundred-miles-an-hour, nose-down, fifty-degree right bank impact with the ground, the captain said to the passengers, "Brace yourself!"

The 727 came down in a residential part of San Diego, killing three women and two boys. None of the occupants of the aircraft survived, making the total death toll 144. Five people on the ground were injured.

The investigators could not agree on the findings. It was generally agreed that the Cessna was difficult to see. Some faulted the Cessna for having changed course; others blamed the controllers, but they were not told that the PSA pilots had lost sight of the Cessna—the approach controller was aware of an automated conflict alert nineteen seconds before the collision but took no action, because alerts were usually nothing of the sort, and he believed the PSA pilots had the Cessna in view.

Regulations were tightened for general aviation aircraft flying into and near major airports, with them obliged to have transponders so that collision avoidance systems work. The FAA installed ILS at Montgomery Field and two other small airports in the county, so San Diego would no longer be used for GA training.

Public Reaction

The crash received much attention. It was the deadliest to date, though only eight months later an even worse one was to occur when a DC-10 crashed at Chicago due to an engine falling off and damaging hydraulic systems controlling the flaps on one wing.

Also, there was a photo of the wounded airliner on fire as shown below.

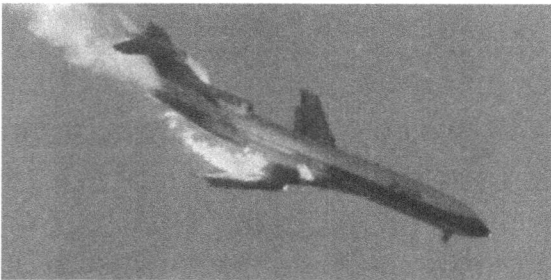

Image taken of PSA Flight 182 by Hans Wendt

Worst-ever Midair Collision (New Delhi, 1996)

Air traffic controllers could not see altitude of aircraft

Delhi had up-to-date radar but had not installed it. Consequently, air traffic controllers had to rely on what pilots told them regarding their altitude and could not see changes in real time.

Kazakhstan Airlines Flight 1907 and Saudia Flight 763, November 12,1996

Besides having archaic radar, Delhi Airport operated under difficult conditions, because the Indian Air Force had appropriated much of the airspace, and both inbound and outbound airliners were funneled along the same narrow corridor, thus greatly increasing the risk of a midair collision.

The midair collision over Lake Constance we describe later in this chapter was similarly in part due to funneling, because the Swiss Air Force had restricted the airspace for civilian flights.

The Saudia (Saudi Arabian Airlines) flight, a Boeing 747-100 with 289 passengers and 23 crew, had taken off at 18:32 local time from Delhi, bound for Dhahran, Saudi Arabia. Coming the other way on its approach to Delhi Airport was a Kazakhstan Airlines charter flight, an Ilyushin IL-76TD, with 27 passengers and 10 crew. Both aircraft were being handled by the same approach controller.

The first-generation Saudia 747-100 had 3 aircrew, 2 pilots and a flight engineer, with the pilots handling communications with air traffic control.

The Kazakhstan Ilyushin had 2 pilots, a captain and first officer, but since it was originally a military aircraft it had a dedicated radio operator sitting at a post behind the pilots without any flying instruments. Handling communications with air traffic control, the radio operator had to lean toward the pilots' shoulders to check the heading and altitude.

Complicating matters further, controllers at Delhi found working with aircrew used to flying only in the old Soviet Union difficult, as they were used to dealing in meters rather than feet, and their understanding of English left much to be desired. Though no one has suggested it, the very fluent but Indian English used by the controllers may not have helped.

Both aircraft were in the same corridor, coming in opposite directions. The Ilyushin wanted to descend to land at Delhi, while the Saudia 747 wanted to climb to its cruising height. To be safe, the approach controller decided to let them pass each other before proceeding.

He therefore allowed the Kazakhstan Ilyushin to descend to 15,000 feet and maintain that altitude and instructed the Saudia 747 to climb to 14,000 feet, leaving a 1,000-foot separation—recognized as being an adequate safety margin.

The Kazakhstan radio operator erroneously reported they were at 15,000 feet when they were not only at 14,500 but still descending.

Even though not in theory necessary, the approach controller warned the Kazakhstan aircraft of the presence of the 747:

Identified traffic twelve o'clock, reciprocal Saudia Boeing 747, ten nautical miles. Report in sight.

He got no reply.

For some reason that has not been established—possibly the pilots misunderstood, bearing in mind they were not talking directly to the controller—the Kazakhstan Ilyushin continued to descend and found itself unwittingly below the 747, when it should have been above it. Even so, although not intended, it should have passed safely underneath.

By a stroke of very bad luck, it was then that the radio operator noticed their altitude was wrong and informed the pilots in no uncertain manner.

The captain applied full power to climb, and as they rose their tail clipped the left wing of the 747, shearing both off. The 747 spiraled downward with the remains of the wing on fire, and the stresses causing it to break up before hitting the ground at over 700 mph.

The Ilyushin did not break up but was uncontrollable, hitting the ground with such force that no one survived, though four people with fatal injuries were found alive.

At that stage in the flight the passengers had probably undone their seat belts. Two passengers strapped in their seats were found alive on the 747 but later succumbed to their internal injuries.

The total death toll was 349.

Aftermath

The shock brought about action that should have been taken long before.

1. The Indian military ceded airspace so that Delhi Airport could have more corridors and never again have incoming and departing aircraft using the same one.

2. Though it took two more years, the languishing radar equipment showing the altitude and identify of aircraft was finally installed.

3. It became mandatory for airliners using the airport to be equipped with TCAS, traffic (alert and) collision avoidance systems.

Any one of these three actions would have prevented the deadliest-ever midair collision.

TCAS—Traffic Collision Avoidance Systems

Systems alerting pilots to the presence of aircraft that could represent a possible danger of collision and if a collision seems imminent order them to take appropriate evasive action—say telling one to go up and the other to go down, and not both to go the same way—are becoming more and more sophisticated.

However, it is essential, and in fact obligatory, that pilots obey TCAS and not the air traffic controller as the following two accounts prove.

Two Japan Airlines Jumbos in Near Miss (Japan, 2001)
Police treat one pilot as a criminal

> TCAS (traffic collision avoidance systems) are now fitted to all airliners to alert pilots of the presence of other aircraft in their vicinity, and, as a last resort, order them to take evasive action in such a way that they turn away and not towards each other. If one of the pilots disobeys, the risk of a collision is increased.
>
> Japan Airlines Flight 907 and 958, January 31, 2001

In terms of the number of lives lost, Japan Airlines holds the record for the worst-ever crash involving a single aircraft.

On January 31, 2001 the airline also almost claimed the record for the worst-ever midair collision. Had the two of its aircraft involved collided, the death toll could have been as high as 677.

Of course, these "records" result principally from the number of passengers packed into the aircraft and not the inherent safety of the airline.

Even so, at the turn of the Century Japan Airlines went through a patch where it was subject to a series of warnings from the Japanese aviation authorities regarding safety. It still had not shaken off the opprobrium poured on it at every opportunity by the Japanese media following the intentional crash with 24 fatalities by a mentally ill pilot as a plane came into land, followed by the deadliest crash ever of JL123, a Jumbo 747.

One reason for the worries of the authorities was a near miss where, following a mistake by air traffic controllers putting two Japan Airlines aircraft on a collision course, the pilot of one of them failed to comply with the TCAS advisory, thereby increasing the likelihood of a collision in what he considered a great feat to save his aircraft. The flights were as follows:

1. **Japan Airlines Flight JL907**, a Boeing 747 with 427 people on board that had just climbed out of Tokyo's domestic Haneda Airport bound for Okinawa to the south and seeking permission to finalize its climb to thirty-nine thousand feet. On board, the flight attendants were just starting to serve drinks.

2. **Japan Airlines Flight JL958**, a DC-10 with 250 people on board coming in from Pusan, South Korea, to land at Tokyo's Narita International Airport, northeast of Haneda Airport.

At 15:46, a trainee controller under supervision duly authorized JL907 to climb to thirty-nine thousand feet (Flight Level 390). Two minutes later the nearby DC-10 crew reported they were at thirty-seven thousand feet (Flight Level 370), meaning their paths would cross in the vertical plane, which of course would not matter if they maintained separation in the horizontal plane.

However, six minutes later the trainee controller discovered they were on courses that could result in a collision. In probably a panicky reaction to the aural warning of the potential conflict, the controller, who had intended to tell JL958 (the DC-10) to descend, mistakenly told JL907 (the Boeing 747) to do so.

The captain of the 747 *descended* in compliance and continued to do so despite his TCAS giving mandatory aural conflict resolution advisories to *climb.*

Meanwhile the TCAS in DC-10 was telling them to descend to avoid a collision.

When the trainee controller noticed the DC-10 not having received having understood he wanted it to descend since he had not used their flight number was continuing to fly level, he ordered it to turn right, but apparently, this message did not get through. The supervisor had tried to order the 747 (JL907) to climb, but in vain, as he said, "JAL 957," which applied to neither aircraft.

Seeing the two aircraft were about to collide head-on, the JAL 747 captain forced his aircraft into an even steeper dive and succeeded in missing the DC-10 by 345 to 550 feet (105 to 165 meters) laterally and between 65 and 200 feet (20 meters and 60 meters) vertically—he passed underneath.

 Drinks trolleys on his aircraft hit the ceiling, and one boy was thrown four seat rows. Five passengers and two crew members sustained serious injuries, while about a hundred crew and passengers sustained minor ones, mostly limited to bruising.

No one was injured on the DC-10, which continued on to Narita as scheduled, while JL907 returned to Haneda Airport with its injured.

To the consternation of many in aviation circles, the Japanese police treated the Boeing cockpit like a crime scene. The captain, who probably thought he had done well to save the aircraft by putting his aircraft into a steeper dive, must have been surprised to find he was going to be put on trial, with prosecutors demanding a custodial sentence, though they subsequently relented.

Prosecutors pursued the air traffic controllers, with at one time a hundred civil service demonstrators protesting outside a court in their favor. Various trials and appeals concerning the air traffic controllers have continued year after year, with one even in 2008.

TCAS

TCAS has proved a very effective tool for preventing midair collisions. Surprisingly, many pilots originally thought it would be a nuisance due to spurious alerts and delayed its introduction.

It alerts pilots to the presence of other aircraft, then the risk of potential conflict, before if necessary ordering mandatory action to avoid a collision. The extra "A" for "alert" is omitted.

There are now improved versions of TCAS that can handle evasive action in the horizontal plane as well as the vertical and tell aircraft to go left or right as well as up or down. If one of the aircraft is ignoring it *and* doing the opposite it can even reverse its instructions.

Distraught Father Assassinates Controller (Lake Constance, 2002)

Only one pilot obeyed the collision avoidance system

> Ironically, had the controller, who was subsequently stabbed to death, not done his best to prevent the collision, it would not have happened.
>
> Bashkirian Airlines Flight 2937 **and** DHL Flight 611, July 1, 2002

One evening a middle-aged stranger came to the suburban residence near Switzerland's Zurich Airport where that air traffic controller, Danish-born Peter Nielsen, lived.

Nielsen had recently returned from medical leave to assume other duties at Skyguide, the Swiss air traffic control company.) After a brief exchange of words at the front door, the unknown visitor proceeded to stab Nielsen to death in full view of his wife.

A senior police officer soon dismissed the notion that it had been a hit man, saying, "Hit men don't get emotional and they don't use a knife."

Soon it was realized that the middle-aged man must have been the father of one or more of the many children killed 623 days earlier in a midair collision over Lake Constance, lying between Switzerland and Germany and touched at its foot by Austria. Many could sympathize but not condone.

The terrible collision had occurred at 35,400 feet in a virtually empty sky at 23:35 local time on July 1, 2002. It had been between a Tupolev-154 airliner with sixty-nine people, including fifty-two children, on board and a DHL cargo plane with just two pilots.

Everyone on the two aircraft lost their lives. Among the dead were the wife, son, and daughter of forty-eight-year old Viktor Kaloyev. Those who knew Kaloyev said he had been implacably distraught since losing everything he had to live for, and, indeed, it was he who murdered Nielsen.

A court subsequently sent Kaloyev to a psychiatric hospital. However, was his act of vengeance misplaced? Was he right to focus on the air traffic controller? As is usual in an air accident, a whole series of unfortunate events and failures, on their own of little consequence, led to the midair collision for which Viktor Kaloyev held Nielsen responsible.

Five and half minutes before the collision, Nielsen had authorized the DHL cargo aircraft, flying north, to climb to thirty-six thousand feet to save fuel. Meanwhile the TU-154 was flying in a westerly direction at the same altitude, meaning they were at right angles.

Their speeds and relative positions were such that they might collide or, rather, risked a lack of separation. Air traffic controller Nielsen would usually have realized this quite soon.

With his companion taking a rest, as allowed by company regulations, outside the control room, Nielsen was handling all the air traffic in the Zurich area.

He had to watch over two screens and slide his chair between them. This would not have been too difficult if traffic had been virtually nil, which was usual at that time of night, or if he had been able to devote all his time to controlling the air traffic rather than placing calls through public phone lines to which he was not accustomed and did not have the special features mentioned.

Also, in the roughly five minutes prior to the collision, he was responsible for four aircraft on one frequency and a fifth on another. Then, moments before the collision, a sixth aircraft called in.

The air traffic control system was in fallback mode for servicing, which meant aircraft needed to be farther apart than usual. In addition, the short-term conflict alert system, which would have warned Nielsen of an impending collision, was not working. It would have given an audible warning and shown the echoes of the aircraft in red. It seems Nielsen was not aware that this was not functioning.

Furthermore, management had allowed engineers to switch off the special phone system, so they could perform overnight maintenance. Though based on quite an old analogue system, it used dedicated lines to link the neighboring control centers, enabling the automatic rerouting of calls if one line failed, and included a priority ringing system so a controller could tell if a call was especially urgent, as in the case in question.

Using unfamiliar public phone lines, Nielsen had wasted considerable time just before the collision contacting a nearby German airport to hand over a delayed incoming Airbus. Worse still, the phone outage meant a controller one hundred miles away in the German Karlsruhe Center who was aware of the possibility of a conflict could not get through to warn him of the danger, despite eleven desperate attempts. Nielsen finally also noted the potential danger of collision, and about forty-four seconds before impact he told the TU-154 to descend immediately, as there was crossing traffic.

The DHL 757 continued to implement the TCAS instructions to descend, but the TU-154, after seeming to have hesitated, obeyed Nielsen instead and also descended. Twenty-two seconds before impact, the TCAS in the DHL 757, sensing the increasing danger, ordered the DHL to increase its rate of descent.

Eight seconds before impact, the TCAS ordered the TU-154 to further increase its rate of climb, though it was descending.

For the occupants of the TU-154, including the many children, death was surely relatively quick. That was not true for the DHL pilots, as their aircraft subsequently flew on relatively intact for some distance and crashed eight kilometers away from the location of the debris from the TU-154, which had broken up in the air. The DHL cockpit voice recorder features the voices of the pilots even after the impact between the two aircraft.

In view of the above, it is difficult to blame Nielsen, who nevertheless found the shock and sense of responsibility difficult to bear. Interviewed by a German magazine two weeks after the accident, he expressed his sorrow but said he was part of a system and networks with many interrelated features even though, as an air traffic controller, he was responsible for ensuring accidents didn't happen.

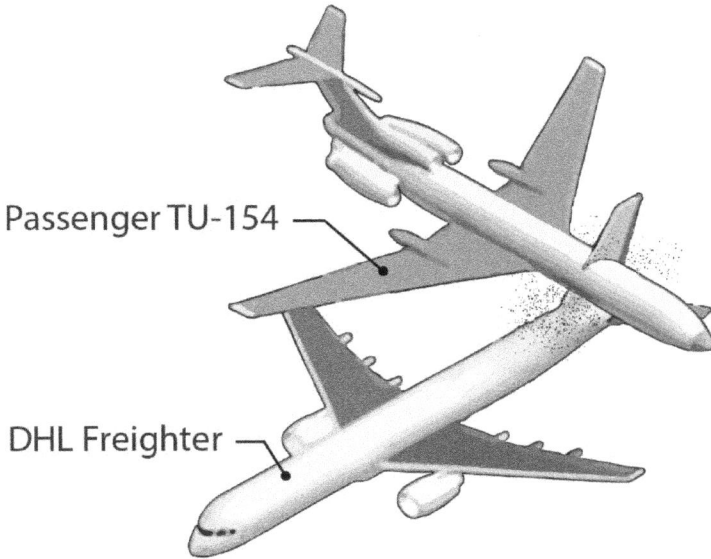

Figurative portrayal based on diagram provided by Germany's BFU

The presence of an extra captain of very great seniority in the jump seat of the TU-154 would seem to have been the tipping factor as regards the failure to obey the TCAS instructions. Apparently, he stopped the first officer doing so, which partly explains the hesitation just mentioned.

The senior captain in the jump seat may have acted thus because he was from the old school and had considerable experience of flying in the Soviet Union, where TCAS is little used and obeying the air traffic controller would be the norm and built into his psyche. Be that as it may, psychologically speaking, after starting to take evasive action by going one way, it is not easy to immediately readjust and switch to doing the opposite.

That said, one must be very unlucky to collide with another aircraft at 11:35 p.m., when there should be a lot of empty space in the sky. One must be even unluckier to collide at right angles, where the horizontal separating effect of any variation in relative speeds is maximal. Some people partly blame the Swiss Air Force for appropriating so much space for itself that commercial airliners are funneled through the rather limited space over Lake Constance.

Though there is a lot of empty sky at night, cargo aircraft, by the very nature of their tasks, often do fly at night. They are especially vulnerable to collisions, because radar systems are taken out of service then for maintenance and everyone tends to be less alert, not only because it is nighttime but also because there is usually not enough action to keep people on their toes.

Sadly, had Nielsen been incompetent or careless and had not finally noticed the potential conflict (lack of separation), the accident would probably never have happened.

All one can say is that he was largely a victim of circumstances, since so much equipment was either in fallback mode for servicing or unavailable, as in the case of the telephones. Regulations and manning levels should not have made it possible for him to be left to cope with everything on his own in such circumstances.

Safer Today

As mentioned in a previous piece, newer versions of TCAS automatically reverse their commands should they find that one aircraft is not complying.

Rate of Descent

It is likely the tail-engine TU-154 trijet, like the Boeing 727 and de Havilland Trident, could achieve exceptionally rapid rates of descent and the TU-154 was dropping must faster than the Boeing 757.

Postscript

Kaloev, the father who killed Nielsen, the controller, was released after two years for good conduct and on mental health grounds. He returned home and was treated as a hero for meting out justice that supposedly had not been done. Indeed, in 2016 he was awarded the highest regional medal by the local Ossetian government, the medal To the Glory of Ossetia.

We must remember many children in that community lost their lives on that holiday trip.

Kaloev was bitter because Nielsen, whom he assumed responsible, was allowed to return to work with no criminal charges at all.

We stand by our account here showing the controller did his best in exceptionally difficult circumstances. In fact, in a way he caused the disaster in trying to prevent it, and the problem was the pilot of one aircraft obeying him and not the TCAS. Had Nielsen not tried, there would... as we have said, been no collision.

Perhaps there is some consolation for Kaloev in that now, aged sixty-two, he has married a woman twenty-two years younger, who in late December 2018 gave birth to a twin boy and girl, with him saying, "Life has turned out so that I have children once more. And I have meaning in my life again. Doctors say that everything is fine with the babies... They were born healthy, everything is fine."

It was a systems and managerial tragedy rather than the fault of the controller and shocked a whole community, but almost unbelievably life goes on.

A 2017 movie, *Aftermath*, with Arnold Schwarzenegger is very loosely based on Kaloev.

Chapter 5
GROUND COLLISIONS

Worst-ever Multi-Aircraft Disaster (Tenerife, 1977)

Strict rules over hours made KLM captain impatient

> A whole series of events led towards this terrible disaster.
> Take any one away and it would not have happened.
> KLM Flight 4805/Pan Am Flight 1736, March 27, 1977

One Sunday afternoon in March 1977, a terrorist bomb and the possibility of another had made the authorities temporarily close Las Palmas Airport in the Canary Islands. Most of the incoming flights were diverted to Los Rodeos, a less important airport on nearby Tenerife, turning that relative backwater into a hive of activity. Aircraft languishing there waiting for Las Palmas to reopen were blocking key taxiways, including the normal parallel route for taxiing to the far end of the runway for takeoff.

Though it had a good, long runway, the airport's ground handling facilities were not designed for aircraft as large as the Boeing 747. As a result, a Dutch KLM 747 and a Pan American 747 parked on the apron were taking up so much of the available space that the Pan Am 747 would not be able to squeeze past the KLM to get out. They were both waiting to resume their journey to Las Palmas.

The KLM 747 had just come from Amsterdam, a four-hour journey, with a group consisting mostly of young Dutch tourists. The 248 people on board included 48 children, 3 babies, 2 pilots, a flight engineer, and 11 cabin crew.

The Pan Am 747 had come from Los Angeles, with a stop in New York for refueling and a change of crew before the eight-hour transatlantic flight to what should have been Las Palmas, where the mostly elderly passengers were to join a cruise liner. The 396 people on board included the 2 pilots, a flight engineer, and 2 company employees in the cockpit jump seats. The 747, *Clipper Victor*, had a dent in its nose made by a champagne bottle striking it to celebrate the inaugural commercial Boeing 747 flight, from New York to London on January 21, 1970. It was one of the first jumbos.

The KLM 747 also supposedly had some fame associated with it, in that a photo of its Dutch captain, van Zanten, was being used in KLM's advertising material, including that in the in-flight magazine the passengers must have been perusing during the long delay. Much has been made of this publicity photo, with suggestions that van Zanten was a self-important stuck-up prig—a captain-of-the-*Titanic*-like figure—as maintained by the Spanish side. The author, as surely were many others, was seduced by this simplistic portrayal until he read *Disasters in the Air*, by Jan Bartelski, a pilot with KLM, who held important posts with the International Federation of Airline Pilots Associations (IFALPA).

Bartelski's role at IFALPA, where admittedly defending the interests of pilots would be paramount, is reflected in his very pro-pilot approach to accidents, but many of the points he makes cannot be lightly dismissed. His thirty years at KLM did also give him some inside knowledge.

According to Bartelski, van Zanten was rather a serious and introverted man, and the only reason for the publicity department using his photo was likely to have been his availability for photo sessions. As a training captain, van Zanten was usually freely available at the home base; other captains would be either away flying aircraft or resting at home. Indeed, the photo of van Zanten included in Bartelski's book gives the impression of a rather accommodating person.

Again, he says van Zanten was not as senior as suggested. It is well known that, because of the influence of powerful unions, much at the major airlines depends on seniority (rather than ability). KLM had promoted van Zanten out of turn to the rank of captain when the captain in charge of 747 training retired, and consequently the Dutch pilots' union insisted he only fly routes when no other captain was available. This limited his amount of line experience even more than normal for a training captain.

First Officer Meurs, also a captain, seconded Captain van Zanten. Though very experienced on other aircraft, Meurs had only flown ninety-five hours on the 747, having shortly before converted to the aircraft under the instruction and authority of Captain van Zanten himself. While this supposedly made Meurs particularly deferential toward him, Meurs was an outspoken and extrovert type, and van Zanten followed his advice at several points while proceeding to the end of the runway for takeoff. Assisting them was Flight Engineer Schreuder.

In charge of the Pan Am 747 was Captain Victor Grubbs, a fifty-seven-year-old with over twenty-one thousand hours of piloting experience. First Officer Bragg and Flight Engineer Warns were with him on the flight deck, together with two company employees in the jump seats.

The waiting dragged on all through the afternoon, with the KLM crew becoming increasingly worried that their permitted flying time would expire. If it did, they would have to stay overnight at Los Rodeos or Las Palmas and fly back to Amsterdam the following morning, upsetting any plans they might have for that day. In the peak season it would be virtually impossible to find overnight accommodation for the passengers.

A number of potential accidents due to fatigue had made the Dutch authorities establish strict legal limits for hours of duty, removing the discretion the captains previously had had in this regard. The regulations were so complex that captains often had to ask the airline's operations center for a ruling to cover themselves. Contacting their HQ by high-frequency radio, the KLM crew was relieved to have a ruling that it would be okay provided the flight back got away before a certain time later that evening.

Finally, with news that Las Palmas Airport had reopened, other aircraft began to take off for that airport, which made Captain van Zanten realize that refueling delays at Las Palmas might jeopardize their chances of getting off from there before their permitted flying hours were up. He therefore opted to refuel at Los Rodeos instead, with enough fuel to continue on to Amsterdam from Las Palmas.

The Pan Am crew found it could not taxi to the runway with the huge KLM jet blocking its path. After the long wait for flights to Las Palmas to be authorized, it was not at all happy to be told by the KLM crew—with no hint of apology—that refueling would take some thirty-five minutes. The Pan Am first officer and engineer got out and paced the ground to see whether there just might be room for them to squeeze by. Visibility was falling, and when refueling had finally finished and the two aircraft could leave the apron for takeoff, it was down to three hundred meters.

Los Rodeos Airport, at an altitude of some two thousand feet, is subject to cloud rather than typical lowland fog. However, it can be quite worrying, as visibility can be very poor at moments and improve or worsen suddenly.

Since the taxiways parallel to the runway leading to the holding point for takeoff were blocked by parked aircraft, the air traffic controller told the two aircraft to enter the runway at the other end and back-taxi up it. The KLM 747 in the lead was to go right to the far end, perform a U-turn, and wait for permission to take off.

The Pan Am 747 was told to follow the KLM 747 but turn off at the third taxiway on the left, to be out of the way and give the KLM a clear runway to take off. As Los Rodeos was merely a diversion airport for emergencies, the Pan Am crew only had a small-scale plan showing the layout. What is more, the taxiways did not have signs identifying them. For the pilots looking at their plan, the obvious exit to take seemed to be the fourth taxiway, since it turned off at a comfortable 45 degrees, with another easy turn onto the main taxiway after that. The third exit, on the other hand, would require two difficult 135-degree turns and initially take them back toward the terminal. Unsure whether the controller had said the first or third exit, the Pan Am pilots had asked him to repeat his instructions. The controller did this, saying, "Third taxiway. One, two, three, third."

On reaching the third taxiway, the Pan Am crew was loath to take it in view of those awkward 135-degree turns, not to mention the additional distance involved, and proceeded slowly onward to the fourth turnoff. Anyway, the controller had told them to report when they left the runway, and it would be inconceivable that he would give the KLM 747 permission to take off before confirming it was clear.

Some commentators have suggested the controller asked the Pan Am to make the awkward 135-degree maneuver because he had little experience of handling aircraft as large as the 747.

However, as the Dutch investigators subsequently showed, this 135-degree turn was by no means impossible. Oddly, no one seems to have suggested that consciously or out of habit, the controller might have been trying to keep the two aircraft well separated in the fog.

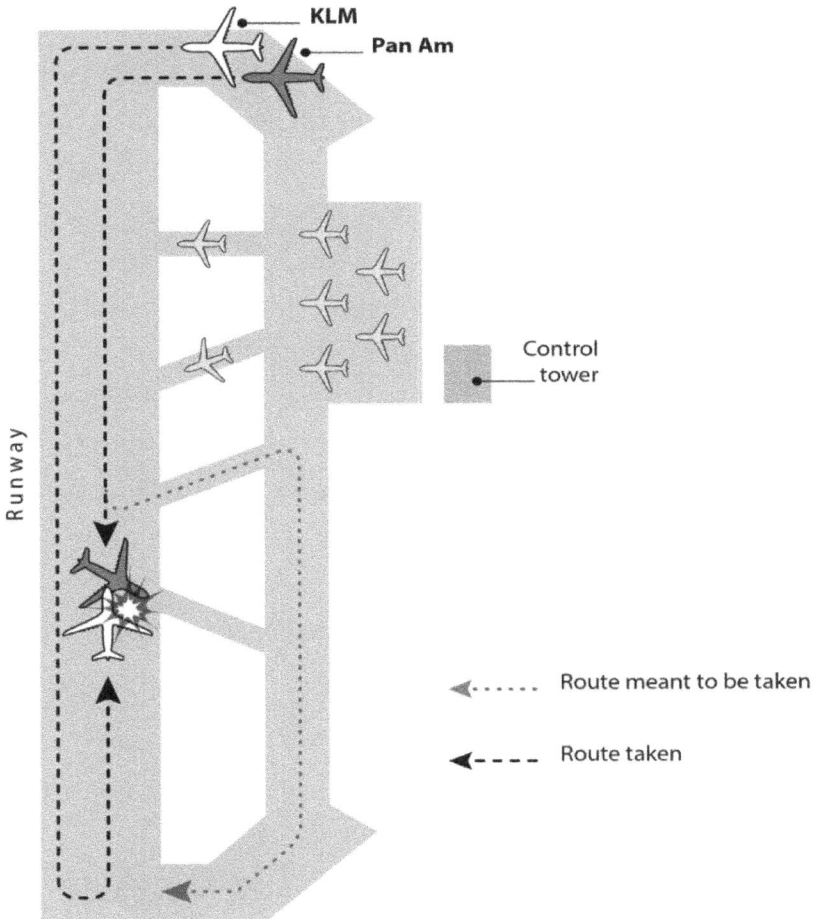

Tenerife's Los Rodeos Airport, now called Tenerife North Airport

Had the Pan Am 747 been instructed to take the fourth and last turnoff and missed it in the poor visibility, it would have come face-to-face with the KLM 747, with hardly any room to maneuver at best. As aircraft cannot go backward on their own, a tractor might have been required to separate them, and this would have meant closing the runway and further delays for all the other waiting aircraft.

On reaching the end of the runway, van Zanten duly made the tight 180-degree U-turn to face back down the runway ready for takeoff, directly facing the Pan Am 747 trundling toward him. The poor visibility meant the aircraft were out of sight of each other and out of sight of the control tower.

Van Zanten spooled up the engines a little and allowed his giant aircraft to inch forward. According to the Dutch comments made later, this application of a small degree of power was a normal maneuver to check the functioning of the engines and not an indication he was about to initiate takeoff. Whatever its significance, First Officer Meurs said:

Wait a minute; we don't have an ATC clearance.

Van Zanten replied:

No, I know that. Go ahead and ask.

He then applied the brakes fully.

Meurs then called the control tower, saying:

KLM4805 is now ready for takeoff—we're waiting for our ATC clearance.

The tower replied:

KL4805. You are cleared to the Papa beacon. Climb to and maintain Flight Level 90. Right turn after takeoff. Proceed with heading 040 until intercepting the 325 radial from Las Palmas VOR.

Van Zanten apparently assumed this meant they were also cleared for takeoff, and as Meurs began confirming the ATC clearance by reading it back to the controller, he released the brakes and this time advanced the throttles to give high, but not maximum, takeoff power.

With Meurs occupied with confirming the ATC clearance, van Zanten then said to Flight Engineer Schreuder:

Let's go! . . . Check the thrust.

The first officer, though preoccupied with reading back the ATC clearance to the tower, added a phrase that could have saved them. However, it failed to do so, because he used a Dutch idiom that in English had a different sense:

Roger, sir, we are cleared to the Papa beacon, Flight Level 90, until intercepting the 325. We're now at takeoff.

Meurs, using the Dutch idiom, meant they were actually taking off, and, indeed, when the two words "at takeoff" left his mouth, the aircraft had already been gaining speed for six seconds. The controller, like anyone used to speaking English, naturally assumed "at takeoff" meant the KLM 747 was at the takeoff position at the end of the runway, awaiting clearance to proceed.

In a run-of-the-mill fashion, the controller then said:

Okay. Stand by for takeoff. I will call you.

However, the crew of the Pan Am 747, feeling vulnerable and fearful that the KLM 747 might take off at any moment, interrupted the tower's reply to the KLM with the frantic words:

We are still taxiing down the runway!

The simultaneous radio transmissions produced a radio squeal called a heterodyne, with the result that the

KLM 747 only heard the single word "okay" from the controller, and not the rest of the controller's sentence or the words from the Pan Am 747 regarding the fact they were still taxiing down the runway. However, the tower did hear the Pan Am transmission and, thinking the KLM 747 was still holding, replied:

Roger, Pan Am 1736, report runway clear.

Pan Am:

Okay, will report when clear.

Controller:

Thanks!

This exchange, which took place when the KLM jet had already been accelerating for twenty seconds, was being followed by KLM Flight Engineer Schreuder, but not by the two pilots, who were concentrating on the tricky takeoff in the fog.

Schreuder expressed his concern to his colleagues somewhat hesitantly in Dutch, with words to the effect of:

Did he not clear the runway then?

Not understanding what he meant, van Zanten said:

What did you say?

The flight engineer clarified his question:

Did he not clear the runway—that Pan American?

Van Zanten and Meurs very affirmatively replied:

Yes, he did.

Having expressed his doubts deferentially as a question rather than as a strong positive statement that the Pan Am 747 was possibly still on the runway, the flight engineer was wrong-footed and merely repeated the questioning statement.

Captain Grubbs, in the Pan Am 747, not knowing that Dutch-speaker Meurs had meant they were actually taking off when he had said "We are at takeoff" nevertheless sensed van Zanten was extremely anxious to get away and might take off at any moment.

Addressing his crew, he exclaimed:

*Let's get the f**k out of here!*

The others agreed, commenting sarcastically about van Zanten keeping them waiting for so long (while refueling) and then developing a sudden urge to get away.

Seconds later the crew of the Pan Am 747 sighted the first glimmer of the KLM 747's landing lights piercing the fog some 580 meters away. Those lights grew brighter and brighter as Captain Grubbs pushed his throttles fully open to try to pull out of the way. He did not stand a chance of succeeding in the eight seconds that remained before the inevitable impact, since his engines needed five of those seconds just to spool up enough to begin accelerating the massive jumbo, with its considerable inertia.

Grubbs and his colleagues could only pray that van Zanten would manage to get off the ground in time to pass over them. One of them even muttered:

Get off! Get off!

It was only as his KLM 747 attained the takeoff decision speed, V_1, of about 140 knots that Captain van Zanten in turn saw the Pan Am 747, which by then was less than five hundred meters ahead of him. Even though he had not quite reached rotation speed, V_R, he yanked the control column so far back that the rear underside of his aircraft made a long gouge in the concrete runway.

Lifting off at that slow speed with the added burden of the 55,500 liters of fuel he had cannily just loaded was never going to be easy. Even so, his aircraft heaved itself up sufficiently for the nose wheel to pass over the Pan Am craft. All to no avail, as the number four engine pod suspended below the right wing struck the Pan Am 747's humped back just behind the flight deck, crushing the first-class upper passenger cabin behind the pilots and ripping off the flight deck roof. When the first officer almost instinctively reached up for the engine fuel shut-off levers, he found nothing there!

Though van Zanten had placed his aircraft in a sharp nose-up attitude, its trajectory at that slow speed and great weight was virtually horizontal. In consequence, the massive main landing gear wheel bogies dangling well below the nose wheel were bound to slam into the roof of the Pan Am's main cabin and crumple it as they rolled over it. Again, that sharp nose-up attitude meant the tail section of the KLM was lower still, so that it in turn sliced neatly between the double tracks of carnage created by the landing gear bogies.

With fire breaking out in both aircraft, the KLM 747 continued its trajectory for a second or two before crashing down onto the runway, with engines and other pieces falling off. After the KLM 747 had slithered to a halt some 450 meters from the point of collision, its fuel tanks exploded, engulfing the fuselage in fire.

None of the 248 people inside the KLM 747 even managed to open a door or emergency exit, let alone jump out.

As already mentioned, passengers usually have a ninety-second time frame to escape when an aircraft on the ground is seriously on fire. In the case of the Pan Am 747, there was only a minute. In the main cabin, where many of the passengers were quite elderly, those still alive on the side opposite the one that received the full impact of the KLM's main wheels had their escape hampered by debris, and few managed to get to the exits.

Helped by the collapse of the floor of the upper-deck first-class cabin behind the flight deck, the three aircrew and the two company staff with them in the jump seats were able to escape, along with those in the lower-deck first-class section below. Those in the upper-deck cabin that had received the direct impact of the KLM's right engine pod did not stand a chance.

A number of the Pan Am passengers had to jump to the ground from a considerable height, sustaining further injury. In fact, nine out of the seventy people who did get out alive subsequently died from their injuries, making the final death toll for that aircraft alone 335.

Adding 335 to the 248 dead in the KLM 747, the total death toll was 583, making it the worst-ever aircraft accident if one excludes 9/11, which largely involved people on the ground.

Conclusion

Had it not been for two things:

> 1. The transmission of the Pan Am saying they were still taxiing down the runway not overlapped that of the tower to the KLM 747 saying, "Okay. Stand by for takeoff. I will call you," so that the KLM only heard "Okay.

> 2. And had the first officer not used the confusing phrase "We are at takeoff," instead of "We are taking off."

the accident might have been averted even at the last minute.

While it has been generally assumed that using the phrase "We are at takeoff" to mean "We are taking off" is quite usual for a Dutchman speaking English, it is possible that the first officer, who was quite used to speaking English, had reverted to using Dutch idiom under the stress engendered by having to read back the airways clearance while the impatient captain was initiating a tense takeoff in fog. One of the US investigators said the voice of the first officer had changed around that time, as if he were stressed or worried. Having stopped van Zanten taking off once because they had not received their airways clearance, perhaps he hesitated to do so a second time and thought he would cover his back by announcing they were taking off—unfortunately, with the wrong choice of words—in which case the controller could tell them to abort if dangerous.

The fact that the KLM aircraft declined, on the grounds of being too busy, to receive that airways clearance earlier meant that Captain van Zanten was preoccupied with handling the aircraft, and the first officer was preoccupied with reading back the clearance. Thus, van Zanten was effectively carrying out a tricky takeoff in fog with help from the flight engineer rather than the first officer.

Flight Engineer Meurs had said, "Did he not clear the runway—that Pan American?" but with the KLM 747 gaining speed he would have had to be much more forceful to get both pilots to back down. Both pilots had unhesitatingly said the Pan Am had.

The Pan Am crew might have made more of the fact in their exchanges with the controller that they were wondering whether they were taking the appropriate exit. However, they did twice indicate they were still on the runway, with their warning on the second occasion doing more harm than good. Perhaps they began to think better of what they had done, and that is why the captain said, "Let's get the f**k out of here!"

The Dutch investigators said the air traffic controller could have performed better and that the sound of a football match being broadcast in the background suggested he might have been distracted from his tasks. Had it not been a critical stage in the match, it is possible the control tower would have made an intermediate check of the Pan Am 747's progress.

Another factor in the disaster may have been that the controllers had been having a grueling day dealing with the many diverted flights, and things were finally easing up, which is just the time accidents tend to happen, as people are a little less sharp once the pressure is off. According to Bartelski, the Spanish authorities very likely sought to protect their controllers by only providing investigators with a poor copy of the control tower recording tape, which could not be synchronized with the cockpit voice recorder (CVR) tapes in the two aircraft.

One point made by Bartelski and not generally known is that following the Tenerife accident, all KLM pilots were made to undergo strict practical hearing tests, and as a result two older captains had their licenses withdrawn. Because of medical confidentiality, Bartelski says, there is no direct evidence that a hearing deficit should be considered as a likely contributory factor. However, he points out that if van Zanten had such a hearing deficit, he would have been more likely to miss the word "report" in that transmission from the tower to the Pan Am 747:

Roger, Pan Am 1736, report runway clear.

Ironically, had KLM not started so rigidly applying regulations regarding maximum flying hours in the name of safety, van Zanten might not have been so impatient.

747 Takes Off on Blocked Runway in Heavy Rain (Taipei, 2000)
Wish fulfillment—you see what you expect to see

> Singapore Airlines (SIA) has one of the best reputations in the industry.
>
> The news of an absurd disaster at Taipei, Taiwan, in which one of its aircraft took off in atrocious weather on a disused runway, came as a great shock.
>
> Singapore Airlines Flight 006, October 31, 2000

An English edition of the Japanese *Yomiuri* newspaper wrote, "In what is probably a world first, the operators of Tokyo's Narita Airport have decided to use paint and nets to camouflage part of the new 2,180-meter runway to keep aircraft from accidentally landing on an unused section. The camouflage is designed to make the superfluous section of the runway look like grass."

Why should Tokyo's International Airport go to so much trouble and expense when all they had to do was to use the traditional X (no entry) signs to denote that section of runway was out of use?

According to officials at the airport, one reason was an incident in 2000, when a Japan Air System jet accidentally landed at Haneda domestic airport on a new but unused runway despite it having those X's.

Another reason may have been the death trap at Taiwan's Taipei Airport into which a Singapore Airlines Boeing 747 was lured on the stormy night of October 31, 2000.

That night one of the worst typhoons that Taiwan was to experience in recent years—dozens of people were killed—was on its way and already bringing torrential rain and gusty winds. If SIA transpacific flight 006, bound for Los Angeles, did not get off quickly, company regulations might forbid it from doing so on account of the increasing crosswind component. Canceling the departure would mean waiting until the crew had its mandatory rest and leaving the next day.

That said, the captain did not seem to be overly hurrying things along to get away before conditions deteriorated further. He apparently told the catering people, who were having trouble loading the victuals due to the terrible weather, to "slow down and take their time." He did, however, take extra precautions, one of which—or as some might say, both of which—were to prove fatal. Firstly, he decided to handle the takeoff himself instead of letting the first officer do it, as had been planned. This meant he would be preoccupied with concentrating on the physical handling of the aircraft rather than on the overall situation.

Secondly, and most unfortunately, instead of choosing Runway 06, on the southern side of the terminal building, which SIA invariably used in view of its proximity to its boarding gate, he opted to use the "safer" Runway 05L to the north. This slightly longer runway should have given a greater margin of safety in the wet and slippery conditions and had the advantage of being a Class II runway, allowing operations in poor weather.

While the captain and first officer had quite often flown out of Taipei, they had not used Runway 05L, on the northern side, for two or three years. The layout they were used to using to the south was much simpler, consisting of just a taxiway and a runway parallel to it.

To reach the main 12,008-foot Runway 05L, they would have to taxi past the end of the shorter 05R runway, which had just been taken out of service (with that end used as a supplemental taxiway), and the middle-to-far end, used to park construction equipment, including concrete blocks.

The trap into which they were to fall was a perfect line of closely spaced green taxi lights leading in a neat curve to disused Runway 05R. In the heavy rain these were very inviting, especially to pilots who were used to Singapore, which has a system whereby controllers turn taxiing lights on and off to show the pilot where to go, so all he or she has to do is to *follow the green*. On the other hand, at Taipei the green taxiway lights leading straight ahead that they should have followed to take them to the operating runway were few and far between, with one not working at all and another quite dim.

Despite the rain and slippery conditions, the SIA 747 captain negotiated the taxiways to the other side of the airport and made the ninety-degree right turn to enter taxiway N1, which would first take them past the end of the narrow disused Runway 05R and then on to the wide, active Runway 05L, which was quite a bit farther on.

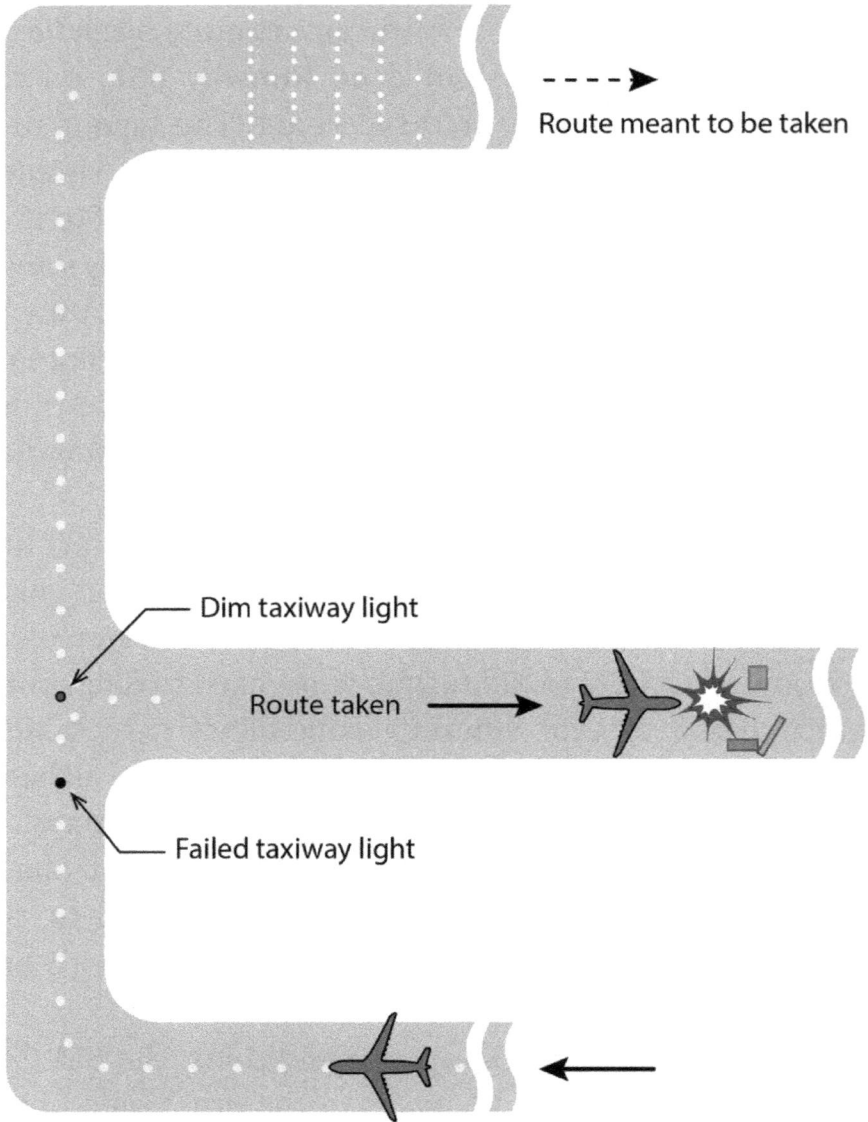

- - - - ►
Route meant to be taken

Dim taxiway light

Route taken →

Failed taxiway light

SQ006 had taxied from southern side of the airport, from where it usually took off

Of course, had visibility been better, the crew of SQ006 would have been able to pick out the bright lights of the operating runway straight ahead.

Indeed, the pilot of a cargo plane belonging to another company that took off eight days after the SQ disaster, but in not quite such poor visibility, said he too had been tempted to follow the bright bright-green lights leading to the disused runway. He had not done so because in the better conditions the bright lights of the operating runway ahead were visible straight ahead.

As every motorist knows, distances seem much greater when moving very slowly in poor visibility, and the crew perhaps thought they had come a fair distance when they mistakenly followed those beckoning green lights and lined up for takeoff from the disused runway. All three pilots assumed it was the runway.

There was a delay of about a minute before they started their takeoff roll, during which it seems they were conscientiously calculating the crosswind component of the headwind to make sure they were not breaking any company rules. Had they not been so preoccupied with the letter of the law, they might have thought it odd the center lights were green and not white, as they should be on an operating runway. It seems—though it is not 100 percent provable—that there were no runway edge lights.

The captain later said he was "80 percent sure" he saw the runway edge lights; the first officer said he did not see any lights other than the center lights. The disused runway was fifteen meters narrower than it should have been, but perhaps the very absence of runway edge lights made this less obvious. Lights shining on raindrops might have given the impression they were difficult-to-see edge lights. On an operating runway there would normally, but not necessarily, also have been the bright touchdown lights, indicating where aircraft should land.

Something the crew did notice and that could have saved the situation was the failure of their para-visual display (PVD) to activate (to unshutter) on turning onto the "runway." The equipment sounds complicated but is merely an instrument with a horizontal rod somewhat like the sign outside a barbershop. A computer senses deviation from the runway centerline and indicates this to the pilots by varying the speed and direction of rotation of the striped rod, producing the optical illusion that the lines are moving to the left or right. This instrument can be helpful for keeping on the runway centerline when visibility is extremely low, even down to fifty meters.

Though this helpful piece of equipment was not working, the pilots did not worry any more about it when they found, on lining up, that visibility was not bad enough for them to need it. After rechecking that the crosswind did not exceed authorized limits, they commenced their takeoff roll. The aircraft gathered pace normally, but four seconds after reaching the takeoff decision speed, V_1, of 142 knots, the captain uttered an expletive and the two words

Something there!

He tried to lift off, but since the aircraft was full of fuel it was too late. Instants later the aircraft's nose wheel hit the first concrete block.

Then, as the huge fuel-laden aircraft was trying to rise, contractors' equipment, including two excavators and a bulldozer, ripped into its hull like the iceberg into the *Titanic*, by which time the speed had reached 158 knots. The 747 fell back, crashed into more construction equipment and concrete blocks, and broke its back. With fire spreading from the left wing, it exploded and ended up, perhaps fortunately, in three pieces.

Some of the passengers and crew were able to scramble out of the breaks in the fuselage and certain exits. Some exits were unusable due to raging fires outside, while the powerful wind made it difficult to open others—some have suggested the Asian flight attendants were not strong enough. In cases where exits could be opened, the escape chutes often did not deploy properly, with one blowing back into the aircraft and pinning down a flight attendant, others flapping around, and some catching fire.

Nevertheless, the survival rate was 54 percent. Of the 179 (159 passengers and 20 crew members) on board, 96 survived and 83 died. Most of the survivors were injured in some way, but as in many terrible disasters, some—16 in all—escaped unscathed. The pilots were among the survivors, and someone saw one of them assisting a flight attendant who had lost a leg.

Big Shock for the Airline

This was a big shock for SIA, an airline highly respected throughout the industry for the expertise of its management and its efficiency.

Except for a crash involving its subsidiary, SilkAir, where there were suspicions that the pilot crashed the aircraft on purpose in a kind of suicide, this was its first fatal crash in its twenty-eight-year history. SIA was also famous for having one of the youngest fleets, at a time when British Airways was still flying some twenty-seven-year-old Boeing 747s.

Many motorists have taken a wrong turning on badly signposted roads in heavy rain, but how could highly trained pilots do such a thing? The captain had 11,235 hours of flight time.

After some bad PR due to their Los Angeles office prematurely reporting no casualties to news organizations phoning from around the world, SIA won plaudits, at least locally, by admitting responsibility, with its chief executive, Cheong Choong Kong, saying at a press conference in Singapore after returning from Taipei, "They are our pilots. It was our aircraft. The aircraft should not be on that runway. We accept full responsibility." In addition, the airline offered to pay $400,000 to the families of those killed and to compensate generously the survivors.

Points Related to This Disaster

A feature of the Boeing 747 that many must have noticed is that the pilots are very high up off the ground, rather like the drivers of some SUVs looking down on others from their lofty perch. The reason for this was that the design for the 747 was originally based on one for a military freighter (the C5A) that could be loaded from both front and rear with large items, such as vehicles.

This height off the ground may have made the task of those SIA pilots seeing the markings on the ground even more difficult. Interestingly, the Airbus 380 design for a true double-deck superjumbo has the cockpit set lower down.

It was quite clear that the taxiing lights at Taipei's international airport left much to be desired. The airport did not have ground radar, which would enable controllers to see the location of aircraft in bad visibility, but Taipei airport is not alone in this regard, and its absence was not contrary to international regulations.

When the Taiwanese authorities finally produced their 508-page report into the disaster, it raised so many points that it was difficult to see the wood for the trees. Many of these points seemed to lay the blame on the SIA pilots rather than the airport. The Taiwanese allowed the Singapore side to participate in the investigative phase, but not in the analysis phase. The Singapore side was unhappy about that and produced a commentary rebutting many of the Taiwanese side's conclusions.

The Singapore view was that it was a systems failure, with many factors involved. The Taiwanese view was that while the airport may have had its shortcomings, the pilots should have, and would have, realized they were on the wrong runway if they had taken more care and paid more attention. Also, according to them, SIA had not trained the captain in poor visibility taxiing.

In some respects, it is paradoxical that the crew may have made the mistake because they were being extra cautious, checking and rechecking the crosswind component to make sure they could take off under company regulations. Unfortunately, their checklist did not include checking repeatedly, and by all possible means, that they were on the correct runway. One could say that the crew should have been trained to consider whether failure of the para-visual display (PVD) to activate (to unshutter) on turning onto the "runway" should be seen as a reason to think they might not be on the active runway, but probably most airlines would have failed to think of that.

One point that might seem strange to some was the Taiwanese Chinese investigators asking the pilots whether they had any cultural problems regarding their relationship with other crew members. This really alluded to the crew being partly Malaysian and partly Chinese.

SIA later dismissed the captain and first officer, after having overtly given them full support during the inquiry. It did not dismiss the third officer even though his facile explanation as to why the para-visual display was not working made them miss an opportunity to realize they were not on an active runway.

Some say this accident was a classic case of scenario fulfillment in that people see what they expect to see.

UK Skyvan Pilots Unable to Follow French ATC (CDG, 2000)

Freighter entered middle of the runway, unaware that...

Shortly before the accident described below, Air France's safety department had recommended its pilots consistently use English in the interest of safety. Not only did some pilots oppose this, but politicians and the press said it threatened the role of the French language in the world.

Air Liberté Flight 8807 and Skyvan freighter, May 25, 2000

It was 02:50 and, with very little traffic, the controllers at Paris's Charles de Gaulle Airport were not using the southern control tower. Besides the usual cargo flights, they had to cope with some twenty thousand Spanish football fans returning to Spain after watching a match between Valencia and Real Madrid in Paris.

Speaking in French, a controller cleared an Air Liberté MD-80 charter flight carrying 150 of those fans for takeoff from the far end of Runway 27. Speaking in English, another controller told the English crew of a Shorts 330 Skyvan cargo plane to hold before entering the second section (3,300 feet farther down) of that same runway, since the small twin-turboprop cargo plane did not need as much runway as the airliner to take off.

The controller had told the crew of the Skyvan that they would be number two. The English captain was wondering who number one was and whether it was the Boeing 737 that had just landed. No doubt thinking that was the case, he moved onto the runway just as the MD-83 was gathering speed on its takeoff run.

In thirty-three seconds, the MD-83 attained V_1 and was just about to reach rotation speed, V_R, when its captain saw the cargo plane nosing onto the runway. With only five seconds remaining before certain impact, he proceeded to abort his takeoff—something virtually never done after attaining takeoff decision speed, V_1. A third of his left wing was shorn off as it struck the nose of the Skyvan, killing its first officer and seriously injuring its captain. With plenty of runway left at such a large new airport, the MD-83's crew were able to bring their damaged aircraft to a halt without any loss of life.

The subsequent inquiry mentioned poor coordination between the controllers, the rainy conditions, and light pollution caused by floodlights and ten vehicles with rotating lights involved in construction work near the threshold. Also, the MD-83 had delayed its takeoff because of an autothrottle problem, and this made the situation evolve rather differently from what the controllers had anticipated.

In addition, it would have been a quiet time, with everyone rather relaxed. Interestingly, psychologists note an inverted U-curve for the effect of stress:

1. No stress; people are not switched on.
2. Medium amount of stress; they are at their best.
3. Too much stress; their interactive skills diminish.

Even so, the key finding apparently was that if communication between the French aircraft and the control tower had been in English, the crew of the cargo plane would have known the MD-83 was about to take off.

Cessna Crosses Runway in Path of SAS MD-11 (Milan, 2001)

Again, failure to use English increased risk of collision

> As usual, this disaster was due to many factors besides the air traffic controllers' actions.
>
> SAS Flight 686/Cessna Citation CJ2, October 8, 2001

Twenty-seven minutes elapsed before the air traffic controllers at Milan's second airport, Linate, realized the two aircraft they had lost contact with had collided at the airport itself.

Milan's Linate Airport is prone to early-morning fog, and at the time of the accident there was no operating ground radar system. The old system had broken down, and the new and much better system bought from Norway some four years earlier had not been set up, due to administrative delays.

After the accident, the so-called administrative and technical problems quickly evaporated, and the system was set up in a couple of months. Part of the delay had been due to an inability to decide whether the airport or air traffic control should be responsible for setting it up.

The brand-new—only twenty-eight airframe hours and twenty cycles—twinjet Cessna Citation, with its two German pilots and two passengers (a Cessna sales manager and a prospective customer) had landed early that morning in fog, with its pilots not qualified to land in such poor visibility.

The Cessna landing in a northerly direction had come to a stop just beyond the taxiway (R6) leading off left to the general aviation apron to the west. However, as there was hardly any traffic at the time, the air traffic controllers allowed it to do a U-turn on the runway and back-taxi to and take taxiway R6, this time to the right. This enabled them to avoid taking a circuitous route via the commercial airliner apron, situated to the northeast.

When they were ready to set off for their next destination, Le Bourget (Paris), visibility was still too bad for the pilots to take off with their pilot's license ratings. However, it was not against the rules for them to taxi in the hope that visibility would improve by the time they were to take off.

Contrary to international convention, the numbering of the taxiways at Linate was not consistent. They should have been numbered in a clockwise direction. R6 should have been R5, and R5, farther around the clock to the north, should have been R6. The Cessna pilots had duly parked on the West Apron after arriving directly from the runway.

However, when it was time for them to leave the West Apron for departure, the airport was busy, so the ground controller instructed them to taxi north via taxiway R5 and call him back when they reached the stop bar to the "main runway extension." Extension was the point on the taxiway in line with the end of the runway that aircraft taking off would overfly.

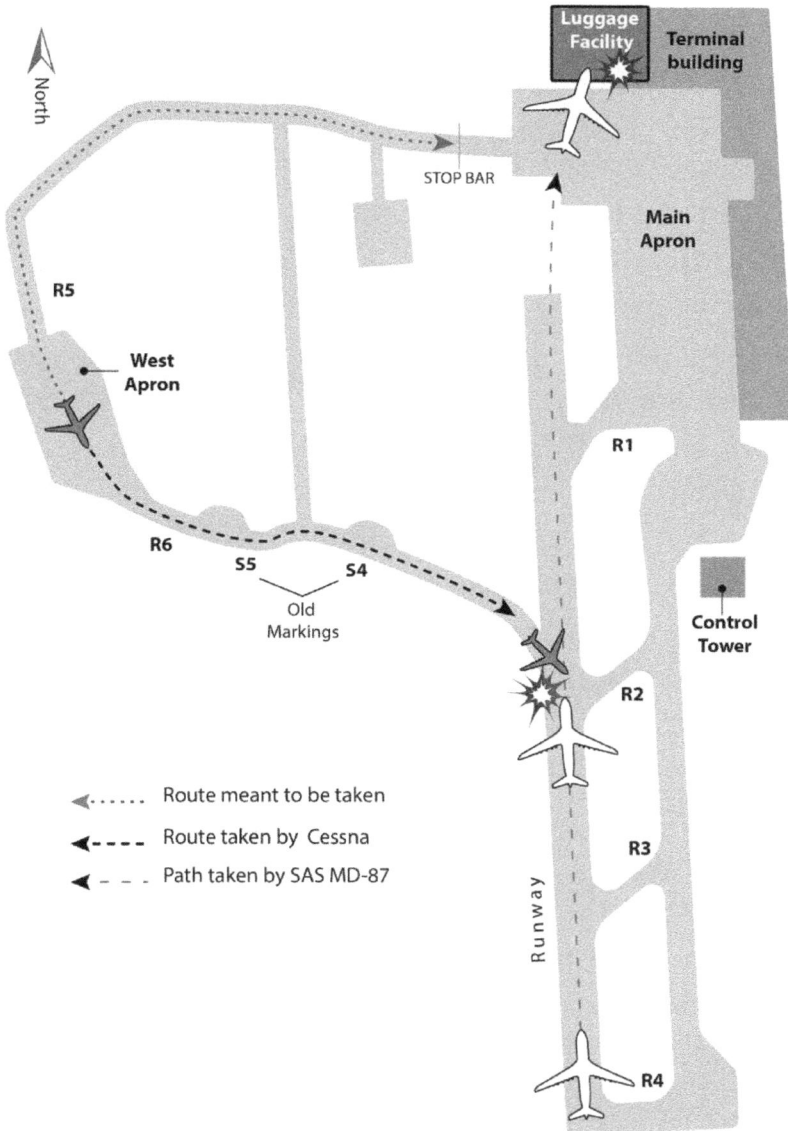

Luggage Facility

Terminal building

Main Apron

STOP BAR

North

R5

West Apron

R6

S5 S4

Old Markings

Control Tower

R1

R2

R3

R4

Runway

⯇······ Route meant to be taken
⯇- - - - Route taken by Cessna
⯇ - - - Path taken by SAS MD-87

Cessna taxied south from West Apron instead of north

Ground control:

DVX taxi north via Romeo five. QNH1013 . . . Call me back at the stop bar at the main runway extension.

DVX:

Roger, via Romeo five and 1013 and call you back before reaching main runway.

The controller did not pick up on the fact that the callback omitted the word "north," but possibly the word was only to make his instruction clearer—for him the pilot had correctly repeated the key information, R5. Some investigators have suggested the German pilot missed the word "north" because it is very short when spoken in English by an Italian.

Seven seconds later the ground controller gave a similar authorization to taxi via R5 to another light aircraft, parked on the West Apron north of where the Cessna had been. However, the controller gave his instructions in Italian and told them to wait until the German Cessna had passed by before moving off. The German pilots in the Cessna could not follow this exchange in Italian.

After a while the controller checked with that second light aircraft, asking them whether they were duly proceeding along taxiway R5. They replied they were still waiting for the Cessna to pass. Their pilot then asked in Italian whether the controller knew where the German was.

The controller replied that the Cessna was on the main apron and added:

I should say you can go.

Frustrated by the unnecessary wait, the Italian pilot replied:

I should say so! We move.

If this exchange had been in English, it might have given the Cessna pilots another hint they were on the wrong track.

The Cessna, erroneously proceeding southeast along taxiway R6 instead of north via R5, came to a spot a little before the runway marked S4 and informed the controller they were "approaching the runway . . . S4."

The controller might have misheard, but the German pilot did use the term "Sierra 4" so it could not have been so unclear. Anyway, S4 did not have any significance. The marking "S4" had been painted on that taxiway many years before when it was thought extra parking spaces might be needed for airliners. However, the project was terminated when the flights were transferred to Milan's other airport. Serving no purpose, it was not mentioned on airport plans used by the controllers.

The controller told them:

Continue your taxi on main apron. Follow the A line.

The Cessna read back the instruction correctly:

Roger, continue taxi in apron, A line . . .

The controller replied:

This is correct. Please call me back entering main taxiway . . .

About that time the controller told an aircraft on the main apron to call back on entering the main taxiway.

The Cessna pilot could have been in no doubt that he was going to cross a (the) runway, but he had the green center lights continuing past the stop bar lights and could have been under the impression that he should cross the runway as quickly as possible.

Having taken the same route in the opposite direction when landing, he should have known he was not at the northern runway extension but possibly in the path of an aircraft taking off or landing.

The Cessna moved forward toward the runway and began to cross, unaware that a SAS MD-87 airliner waiting to start its takeoff roll had received its takeoff clearance and was already moving forward. They were unaware of this fact, as the takeoff clearance had been, as is normal, on the tower frequency, which the taxiing Cessna pilots would not be using.

The point where the Cessna was traversing the runway proper was one and half kilometers from the point where the SAS aircraft had started its takeoff roll just thirty-seven seconds earlier. Consequently, the SAS MD-87 was traveling at about 146 knots and well into its rotation when it encountered the Cessna directly in its path.

The nose landing gear lifted off two seconds before the impact, and though the main landing gear was still touching the ground, the weight was coming off the main wheels, with their shock absorbers extending. (The liftoff of the nose wheel had automatically sent a signal to the SAS home base in Copenhagen indicating that the flight had duly taken off!)

A fraction of a second before impact, there was a distinct nose-up elevator input and crew exclamation on the MD-87, so they could only have seen the tiny Cessna at the very last moment. Following the collision, the crew of the MD-87 advanced the throttles farther, but the extra power from the engines mounted at the rear was not forthcoming, as the right-hand number two engine had fallen off and the only remaining engine was failing, no doubt due to ingestion of debris.

Nevertheless, the MD-87 continued its climb to a height of ten and half meters (thirty-five feet) before plunging down onto the runway eight and half seconds after separating from the Cessna. Not only did the MD-87 not have enough thrust from the remaining engine to climb away, the loss of the heavy, rear-mounted number two engine meant the center of gravity had moved too far forward for the aircraft to fly. Realizing the hopelessness of the situation, the pilots pulled back the throttle levers.

Having vainly accelerated to a speed of 166 knots, the MD-87 hit the runway, with the right-hand main wheels missing and failing hydraulic pressure. This meant that the aircraft tipped to the right and the right wingtip struck the ground, causing the aircraft to slew around. The crew adroitly applied reverse thrust to the remaining left-hand engine, but with the tail-mounted engine so close inboard, unlike those mounted engines mounted far out on the wings, the directional correction it provided was limited.

Added to that, lack of hydraulic pressure meant the brakes were ineffective. Veering slightly to the right, the SAS MD-87 was still traveling at 139 knots when it slammed into the luggage-handling building located 460 meters beyond the end of the runway and not far to the right of the runway axis. Just six seconds had elapsed from the moment the MD-87 fell back on the runway and its collision with the building.

Four baggage handlers in the building, and all 104 passengers and 6 crew on the airliner, were killed.

The situation for the two pilots and two passengers in the frail Cessna was hopeless from the start, and all were either immediately killed by the impact or within a minute or so by the fire and smoke. All told, the death toll was 118. Had it not been for the fine airmanship of the MD-87 crew in trying to straighten out the trajectory, it could have been even worse, with the aircraft veering farther to the right and striking the passenger terminal.

Analysis

As mentioned at the beginning of this section, the failures of the controllers and those running the airport were so many and so glaring that they were held criminally responsible. However, did the investigators fully consider the possible fatigue of the Cessna pilots?

The official report only said they presumed the Cessna pilots' duty time had started at 04:30 local time. One supposes they worked this out from the time it would have taken the pilots to fly to Linate from Cologne.

One of the German pilots was sixty-four and the other thirty-six. There is no knowing what they were doing before they picked up the aircraft for the middle-of-the-night departure from Cologne, but it is quite likely they would have been pretty tired by the time they asked for clearance to taxi at 06:05 at Linate. That was the moment they made the fatal mistake of not noticing the air traffic controller had said they should go *north* and call him back when they reached the stop bar at the main runway extension.

What the controller quite meant by "*runway extension*," may not have been clear. Since the Cessna pilots did not confirm the word "*north*," they possibly had not noted it. It is quite possible that after their brief break, one or both German pilots were not fully alert. Without evidence from a cockpit voice recorder, it is difficult to be sure of the exact situation; they could have been distracted by the passengers' presence.

Nevertheless, how the Cessna managed to take taxiway R6 instead of R5 is something of a mystery, unless one assumes that the pilot looking at the plan of the airport was not concentrating, because of tiredness or some other reason. It was confusing, if not looking at the plan, to have taxiway R5 after R6 in the clockwise direction. In addition, as they had followed that route on coming off the runway on their arrival, that route might have seemed more logical, as it was only about a third of the distance to the point where they would start their takeoff.

There is a slight parallel with the crew of the Pan Am 747 at Tenerife in that their taking the easy taxiway at 45 degrees, rather than the difficult one at 135 degrees leading back toward the terminal, would seem more logical and be much shorter.

The Cessna pilots only had one chance to determine what number taxiway they were on, and that was where the yellow lines on the apron forked, with the yellow line for taxiway R5 forking to the left (and north), and the yellow line for taxiway R6 forking to the right. The nearest taxiway light in the direction of R6 was only 80 meters away, while that for R5 that they should have taken was 350 meters away, thus perhaps luring them in the wrong direction, just as with the Singapore Airlines pilots at Taipei. However, if the Cessna pilots and the Singapore Airlines pilots had been looking at the plan of the airport, they surely would have seen their error.

Once the Cessna pilots made the mistake—for whatever reason—there was no further indication along the whole length of the taxiway R6 giving its number. Whatever the truth, the controller pigeonholed them in his mind as being on R5, and nothing they said, apart from the meaningless (to him) statement that they were at S4, suggested otherwise. Even if they missed the stop bar on taxiway R5 at the runway extension, the controller would assume they could not come to much harm, as any aircraft taking off should be well into the air by then.

Chapter 6
CONTROL SYSTEMS
COMPROMISED

DC-10 Cargo Door Opens Inflight (Windsor-Detroit, 1972)

Reinforcing cabin floor for a piano saved the day

> Systems operating essential airfoils (ailerons, elevators, rudder, etc.) are usually in triplicate, and the chance of them failing of their own accord is minimal. The hydraulic power they usually require is provided in most cases by two, or more often three, circuits.
>
> However, if the cabin floor buckles, the hydraulic lines attached underneath can rupture, damaging all three, making the aircraft impossible to control.
>
> American Airlines Flight 96, June 12, 1972

On June 12, 1972, an American Airlines DC-10 bearing flight number 96 took off from Detroit for Buffalo with only fifty-six passengers. Normally, there would have been no need to open the rear cargo hold with so little baggage to load, especially as they would not want to shift the center of gravity too far back. However, the manifest included a coffin, and perhaps out of consideration for the baggage handlers at Buffalo the decision was taken to load it into the rear hold, situated under the floor of the aft passenger cabin.

Though the point of departure and the destination were both in the United States, the route was almost entirely over Canada, as the frontier came southward to follow the center of Lake Erie. With the first officer at the controls and flying on autopilot over the Canadian side of the lake, they were near Windsor, Ontario, and coming up to twelve thousand feet on their routine climb to twenty-three thousand feet when the pilots heard a bang from behind and felt the impact of a rush of air on their faces. The flight deck door sprang open, and a lot of dust started flying around. An explosive decompression had occurred.

Back in the passenger cabins, the rush of air was propelling papers and other loose items rearward, with the situation being worst right at the back, where two flight attendants in seats by the rear doors were for a moment sucked downward toward the floor, buckling into the cargo hold below. The flight attendant on the left could peer into the cargo hold and see the gaping black hole where the door had once been.

Unaware of this, the pilots' immediate thought was that something had struck them, but whatever the cause of the decompression, they first had to determine what controllability they had:

1. The rudder pedals were jammed against the stops at the full-left-turn position.

2. All three throttles had sprung back to their idle stops.

3. Engines one and three, mounted on the wings, seemed to be okay and, despite having begun to spool down due to the movement of the throttles, responded when these were pushed forward.

Engine number two in the tail was no longer functioning and its throttle was immovable.

4. The vital (apart from the rudder) control surfaces in the tail, namely the elevators, were barely working and felt very heavy.

5. Despite the rudder pedals being jammed at full left, the rudder itself angled to the right was making the aircraft yaw to the right. However, by increasing the power on the right engine, reducing that on the left engine, and applying a fair amount of left aileron to make the aircraft bank to the left, it was possible to get it to fly relatively straight.

Subsequently, by adjusting engine power and varying the amount of aileron, the pilots found they were able to steer the aircraft very roughly where they wanted to go, with an inevitable time lag between the input and the response due to the engines needing time to spool up and down.

The DC-10 is notable for having the engines mounted under the wings and very low slung, with this compensated for by having the engine in the tail very high up and at a slight angle. This leverage allowed the pilots to raise or lower the nose by juggling engine power. However, without the compensatory engine high up in the tail, there was a danger of pushing the nose up too far and not being able to push it down. The pilots had to be very wary and proactive—if they got into too sharp a dive, they might not be able to pull out of it, or in trying to do so might not be able to push the nose down afterward and end up stalling.

By making a long, shallow approach, the captain managed to bring the aircraft down onto Detroit's runway, which was 10,500 feet (3,200 meters) long and 200 feet (60 meters) wide, at just thirty knots over the normal approach speed and even managed a flare by having both pilots heaving back on the leaden elevator controls at the last moment.

The touchdown was a good one in the circumstances, but once they were on the runway, application of left aileron could not prevent their trajectory veering to the right, because of the rudder sticking out to the right. As they left the runway, the first officer, realizing they would be in trouble before the reverse thrust and brakes could slow them enough, increased reverse thrust on the left engine beyond the normal limit and at the same time disengaged reverse thrust on the right-hand engine by pushing the throttle lever forward. This succeeded in countering their deviation, and it was not long before their airspeed had dropped enough for the protruding rudder to have little effect, so that the nose-wheel steering, always wanting to veer left under the command of the jammed rudder pedals, came into play, bringing the aircraft back to the runway. They ended up half on and half off the runway, and some five hundred meters from the end.

The captain had not jettisoned fuel, because of uncertainty regarding the extent of the damage to the rear of the aircraft. Even had he opted to do so, the fuel dumping limitation (already mentioned) on the DC-10 would not have allowed him to drain the tanks enough to prevent fire in a crash landing.

The few occupants were able to evacuate in less than a minute, making it a lucky outcome for all concerned. Proficient handling of the stricken aircraft by the crew had saved the day, but why had the incident happened in the first place, and why did the apparent failure of a cargo hold door have such consequences?

The simple answers are:

1. The door-locking mechanism was badly designed.
2. The floor did not have vents in it to allow air to pass through it without it buckling first.
3. The control lines for the rudder, elevators, and rear engine were attached to the underside of that floor.

It so happened that the cabin floor had been specially reinforced to support a piano for some event. Otherwise, it would have no doubt crumpled further, as was to occur a couple of years later to a fully laden DC-10 that had taken off from Paris (See next account).

The Door-Latching Mechanism

Recovery of the cargo hold door from a field under the flight path meant the investigators had all the elements required to determine the immediate cause of the near disaster. The hinges and interfaces between the door and the fuselage were all in good condition, and the investigators quickly concluded the C-latches must have opened for some reason.

As their name implies, the C-latches affixed to the bottom of the door are shaped like the letter C, and in theory they swivel around when the door is locked so as to encircle a very solid crossbar (spool) on the doorjamb, so that the greater the force trying to prize the door open, the firmer it should hold. This supposes proper engagement of the C-latches in the first place.

Unfortunately, the give in the various levers and components of the locking mechanism, and poor design, meant those doors on DC-10s could appear to be locked when in fact the C-latches were not properly home. This was partly because the original design had envisaged using hydraulic power to operate the primary (nonmanual) locking system, and this was subsequently changed to electric on the demand of the airlines on grounds of economy (cost and weight). Hydraulic operation is generally much more positive.

McDonnell Douglas

McDonnell Douglas, the DC-10's manufacturer, had had numerous complaints from airlines about the door in question. The problem with the aft cargo hold door and some other early problems with the DC-10 were said to be due to the frenetic pace at which the aircraft was brought into production, with Lockheed's very similar TriStar in direct competition, and the Boeing 747 lurking in the background.

Although the competing Lockheed TriStar L1011 was an excellent aircraft, McDonnell Douglas had the advantage that US airlines were so used to buying its aircraft that they were likely to choose them out of habit and inertia. This did not prevent the airlines playing off the two companies against each other, with the result that prices became so low that neither aircraft would ever be a big money-spinner, unlike the Boeing 747, which was in a category above.

In addition, delays in developing the power plant for the TriStar had almost led to the demise of the UK engine manufacturer Rolls-Royce, which had to be bailed out by the British government, and in turn meant that Lockheed got off to such a delayed start that sales never took off. Despite offering inducements (bribes) to sell the aircraft abroad, total sales only came to some 250 units, compared with the 500 needed for the project to break even. This ultimately led to the great Lockheed, famous for airliners as the beautiful Constellation, withdrawing completely from the civilian airliner market.

Inducements paid in Japan in the expectation that All Nippon Airways (ANA) would purchase the TriStar led to the resignation and subsequent trial of the Japanese prime minister, Tanaka Kakuei. In parallel, a very senior manager at Hong Kong's Cathay Pacific Airways had to resign in disgrace for accepting inducements, albeit on a much smaller scale.

Ironically, the two did their respective airlines a favor by stopping them from jumping on the dangerous DC-10 bandwagon before its problems were resolved. The DC-10 that crashed outside Paris, as described in the next narrative, with the loss of all on board had originally been destined for Japan's ANA!

Like the fatal *"put on your manager's hat"* decision to launch the Challenger Space Shuttle, many engineering ethics courses cite as classic examples for study the decisions subcontractors made concerning the DC-10 cargo hold door, when engineers were fully aware of the problems.

The Subcontractors

The contractor for McDonnell Douglas was Convair, and six weeks after the Detroit/Windsor incident in 1972, Convair's director of product engineering, Daniel Applegate, submitted a memo to his superiors officially delineating problems with the cargo hold door, which had become apparent as early as August 1969. These had been confirmed in a ground test the following year. According to some reports, those tests also revealed what could happen to the passenger cabin floor.

Following the discovery of the problems by its engineers, Convair's management was halfhearted in pursuing the matter with McDonnell Douglas for fear that under the terms of its contract it might have to pay the cost of the modifications. McDonnell Douglas's management was in turn fearful about the effects any delay might have on its sales. Undoubtedly, the best option would have been to redesign the whole thing, but as such systems have to go through a lengthy approval process with the FAA, it was too late to start over, and it therefore fiddled with an "approved" design, as modifications would only be minor and quickly certified. (Another instance where regulations meant to ensure safety have the opposite effect.)

The opening of a cargo hold door at altitude is always a serious matter, as the slipstream usually wrenches it off. If it is a front cargo hold door, it could damage the control surfaces on the wings or disable the engines under the wings or, if at the rear, damage the horizontal stabilizer and elevator on the tail, as happened in the Detroit/Windsor case.

What manufacturers did not properly consider at the time was the disastrous knock-on effects of such a decompression. Not only would the passengers' risk being sucked out or struck by flying objects, they would also be subjected to the physiological effects of explosive decompression. The downward buckling of the passenger cabin floor under the pressure differential could also damage the vital control links and hydraulic lines leading to the tail, generally attached to its underside. This in turn could make the aircraft uncontrollable.

Within three weeks of the Detroit/Windsor scare, the NTSB made two urgent recommendations:

1. Modification of the DC-10 door-locking mechanism so that it is physically impossible to bring the vent-flap-locking handle to its stowed position without the C-latch locking pins being fully engaged.

2. Vents (holes) should be incorporated in cabin floors to greatly relieve sudden pressure differentials, such as those caused by the opening of a cargo hold door in flight.

The Gentleman's Agreement

The NTSB could only advise. It was up to the FAA to make these two modifications mandatory.

Just when the FAA was about to issue an airworthiness directive (AD) making interim and long-term solutions mandatory for all US operators of the DC-10 (which foreign operators would have followed), discussions between the FAA administrator and the president of the Douglas division of McDonnell Douglas led to the senior FAA technical staff being overruled. Douglas and the FAA were no doubt being subjected to pleading from US airlines, who would not want to take their aircraft out of service in the peak summer season. So, the FAA did not issue that airworthiness directive. Instead, McDonnell Douglas almost immediately issued recommendations, in particular the installation of a "lock mechanism viewing window."

This gentleman's agreement between the FAA administrator and McDonnell Douglas's Douglas division president sufficed to prevent a repeat accident *in the United States*, but not overseas, as the following sad account will show.

DC-10 Cargo Door Again Opens Fatally Inflight (Paris, 1974)
A carbon copy of the previous incident, but deadly

> This DC-10 crash outside Paris was a rerun of the Detroit/Windsor incident, but without the passenger cabin floor having been reinforced for a piano.
>
> Turkish Airlines Flight 98, March 3, 1974

Demand that day for seats between Paris and London was particularly high, as one of the two main airlines serving the route, British European Airways (BEA) crew members were on strike.

This movement was part of a negotiating tactic to get a better deal for BEA staff in its merger with British Overseas Airways (BOAC), to form what is now British Airways (BA). There was some friction, as BOAC people appeared to see themselves superior to those at BEA, who were apparently paid less to fly not-so-exotic routes.

Fans returning to England from a rugby match in Paris the previous day were putting added pressure on the few available seats.

Hence when a Turkish Airlines DC-10 arrived en route for London, stranded travelers clamored for seats, and as a result it departed for London with most seats filled, which was unusual. Taking off in an easterly direction from Orly Airport, situated to the south of Paris, it skirted the city and continued some twenty-five miles before turning north toward England, with everything seeming routine.

Just as the almost-full-to-capacity wide-bodied DC-10, was climbing to cruising height and came abreast of the northern limits of Paris's suburbs at a height of some nine thousand feet and a speed of three hundred knots, the Detroit/Windsor DC-incident replayed itself. However, this time the floor had not been reinforced and so opened up much more. Six hapless—or perhaps fortunate—passengers were sucked downward and disappeared through the chasm in the floor and out of the failed door to subsequently hit the ground still strapped-in in the two rows of their three-abreast seats.

Coinciding with an emergency transmission from the aircraft, French air traffic controllers saw flight number 981 transmitted by the DC-10's transponder disappear from the secondary radar. However, the primary radar, which works by bouncing a radio wave off an aircraft, showed the echo separating into two blips: a large one and a much smaller one. The large one veered northwestward before disappearing after a minute, while the weaker one representing the six passengers in their seats no doubt held together by the broken-off rail used to attach the seats to the floor remained at the same location before disappearing after a couple of minutes or so.

The large blip (the aircraft itself) had come down in Ermonville Forest, some *thirteen miles* northwest of the point where the decompression had occurred. The high sink rate and forward speed meant the trees could not cushion the terrible impact.

Air crash sites are usually horrible, but this one was particularly so. The absence of a conflagration meant the scattered distribution of body parts was immediately obvious.

In *Air Disaster: Vol. 1*, Macarthur Job says how Police Captain Lanier, who was one of the first to arrive, described the terrible scene and saw two severed hands, a man's and a woman's, clasped together. In such circumstances, there was no hope of any survivors.

The Pilots

What had been the situation on the flight deck in those final minutes? Could the pilots have saved the aircraft? Indeed, it seems they had finally found a way to at least bring the aircraft out of its fatal plunge but did not have enough height left. The buckling of the floor had, as in the Detroit incident but to a greater degree, damaged or severed the triplicate hydraulic lines serving the tail and the control cables both for the tail flight-control surfaces and rear engine.

From the cockpit voice recorder (CVR) and the flight data recorder (FDR), investigators ascertained that pressurization-warning klaxons sounded in the cockpit when the cargo door blew out and that the crew thought there had been a failure of the fuselage. Not that it made any difference in this case. Apparently, the situation developed as follows.

As the DC-10 went into a twenty-degree dive, its airspeed increased alarmingly, and despite the engines being throttled back, the overspeed alarm sounded.

With not quite a minute having elapsed since the nightmare started, the captain astutely decided their only hope was to ignore the aural overspeed warnings and go for even more speed. Pushing the throttles forward, he said, "*Speed!*"

Whether it was the speed itself or the nose-raising torque of the two viable engines slung so low below the wings, or a combination of both, the aircraft gradually began to level out, with the rate of descent decreasing so much that the g-forces would have forced the pilots and passengers hard down into their seats. They were almost level when they struck the trees of Ermonville Forest at 430 knots. Had they had a greater height margin, the story could have been different, with the captain's call for speed allowing them to fight on.

All 339 people remaining on board died in the subsequent crash. Perhaps because the captain had cut the engines just before impact there was no major outbreak of fire.

As the high-speed impact had so traumatized the bodies, it was evident that this absence of major fire would not have made much difference to the occupants. However, the relative lack of smoke and fire did make it surprisingly difficult to locate the exact site of the crash in the relatively vast forest. The total death toll, including the six passengers ejected earlier, came to 345.

Comparison

With so little means of control—just the engines—the situation facing the Turkish pilots was more akin to that faced by those of the Sioux City DC-10 than that at Detroit.

However, in the Paris case, only seventy-two seconds elapsed between the decompression and impact with the ground, and only ten seconds between the initiation of the almost successful addition of power to bring the aircraft out of its dive and that impact. Had the Paris pilots been able to recover in time, would they have been able, or lucky enough, to replicate the Sioux City feat?

With the aircraft having disintegrated into tiny pieces, as had the passengers, it looked as if the investigation would be difficult. Postmortems of the relatively intact passengers ejected right at the beginning in their seats provided valuable evidence, and, notably, indicated that the crash was not due to a bomb, as had first been feared. Furthermore, recovery of the cargo door with its mechanism virtually intact, as in the Detroit/Windsor case, was a great help. The investigators found:

1. The stiffening of the linkage from the flap handle had not been done as prescribed in Service Bulletin 52-37. Some modifications had been made, but an item not up to aeronautic quality had been used, and in fact this had made the door even more vulnerable to improper locking than the one on the Detroit DC-10.

2. The microswitch system for indicating (in the cockpit) whether the door was locked was not adjusted optimally.

3. The door did have the prescribed window for checking whether the latches had gone home, but the cargo handler responsible for closing the door was not qualified or told to perform that check.

This was normally done by a Paris-based Turkish Airlines engineer, who was on holiday, or in his absence by the flight engineer, who failed to do so.

The gentleman's agreement between the head of the FAA and the president of the Douglas division of McDonnell Douglas had meant the radical measures recommended by the NTSB after Detroit were not made mandatory. Even the half measures proposed by McDonnell Douglas's Service Bulletin to airlines had not been carried out on an aircraft ordered and delivered long afterward. Three engineers at Douglas or its subcontractor had signed them off as done!

The airline and the manufacturer paid out some of the highest compensation ever for an air disaster, without admitting culpability.

Though the main problem was one of engineering ethics, there were, as usual, multiple factors, including the fact that the flight engineer did not do a visual check through the observation window prior to departure from Paris. The FAA hurriedly made the measures the NTSB had recommended mandatory. These included floor vents. Passengers are safer now thanks to that.

DC-10's Textbook Speed Seals Fate of AA191 (Chicago, 1979)

Would not have flipped if flying slightly faster

> The photo of the DC-10 banking at ninety degrees with one engine missing told all. An engine had fallen off the wing.
>
> American Airlines Flight 191, May 25, 1979

J ust as the American Airlines DC-10 afternoon flight taking off from Chicago for Los Angeles was rotating at a takeoff decision speed (VR) of 145 knots, the rear support of the pylon holding the number one (left) engine failed.

The powerful takeoff thrust then pushed the engine assembly forward and upward as it pivoted on the front support, which in turn fractured. Finally, the engine, with the pylon still attached, passed over the top of the wing and, because of its weight and the low airspeed, tumbled to the ground without damaging the DC-10's high-up tail assembly. The wing minus its engine dipped for a moment but then came up again as the pilot used the ailerons to climb out at 159 knots—6 knots above the minimum climb-out speed (V_2).

Despite the separation of the engine, there was every indication they would be able to return safely to the airport, and the controller observing the takeoff from the tower asked the pilots if they wanted to come back, and if so on which runway.

According to the flight data recorder (FDR), the aircraft then accelerated, reaching a maximum speed of 172 knots nine seconds after becoming airborne. At 140 feet agl (above ground level) and still climbing, the pilot apparently let the airspeed fall back, in accordance with the airline's engine failure procedure.

On reaching a height of about 325 feet, with the airspeed dropping back to the recommended 159 knots, the left wing from which the engine had fallen inexplicably began to drop. The aircraft yawed to the left and was soon sideslipping in a ninety-degree bank, with the wings perpendicular to the ground, as shown in the photo on the next page.

The final reading, obtainable from the data recorder three seconds prior to the left wingtip hitting the ground, showed 112 degrees' bank and a nose-down attitude of 21 degrees. The aircraft then flipped over and exploded, and a large fireball engulfed the debris.

Would-be rescuers said the crash scene was a horrible sight, with no bodies intact and even the remains charred beyond recognition. All 271 people on board were killed, together with two bystanders, making it the worst air disaster up to then in US history.

It could have been worse, as the aircraft came down just short of a large caravan park, and there were fuel storage tanks farther on.

For the hundred or so investigators sent to the scene, there were two main questions:

1. Why had the pilots lost control when the aircraft should have been able to fly in that configuration at that airspeed?

2. Why had the engine and pylon fallen off in the first place?

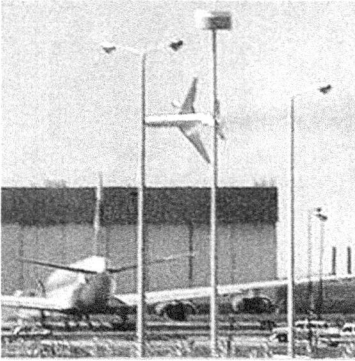
(Courtesy NTSB)
Left wing stalls as slats on that wing retracted

Change-of-Configuration Stall

The outer leading-edge slats on the left wing had for some reason retracted, and this had led to a change-of-configuration stall—that is, a stall where an alteration to the position of the flaps and/or leading-edge slats means the aircraft can no longer fly at the given airspeed.

Paradoxically, had the captain not followed the rule book to the letter and reduced speed on the loss of the engine, he would have been above the stalling speed for that configuration, and the ailerons would have been sufficient to compensate for the discrepancy in lift due to the retracted outer slats on the left wing. He could have flown all the way to Los Angeles.

The rule (later modified) had been made to protect the other engines, which automatically spool up to maximum or above maximum rated power when an engine fails on climbing out on takeoff to compensate for the loss of power. The pilots are told they should level out and decrease the power on the remaining engines, which the pilots of the DC-10 duly did.

However, as in so many crashes, there were other unfortunate factors. Firstly, on twisting upwards and skidding over the wing the engine assembly had severed a cable passing just inside the damaged leading edge of the wing that should have transmitted the information that the slats had retracted to the pilots.

Secondly, the stick shaker (stall warning system) did not activate, and the instruments were not working properly because the electric circuit had been locked out. Also, with the inner slats still deployed there would have been virtually no buffeting that the pilots could sense. That electrical system could have been unlocked by the pilots, but they were too busy, and for the engineer to do so, he would have had to turn his seat around and unbuckle himself, which was hardly possible in the time available.

Not knowing what was happening, and with no time, the pilots could not have been expected to realize where the route to salvation lay. Also, the dissymmetry in lift and resultant banking meant that the minimum control speed (V_{MC}), as well as the stalling speed, would rise so quickly that even getting the wings level would quickly become hopeless.

Pilots given the full background were able to save the aircraft in the simulator, but those not so briefed reacted as the actual pilots had and crashed.

DC-10 Design

The DC-10, unlike many other aircraft, did not have a mechanical locking device to keep the slats from retracting under external force in the event of a failure. However, in most cases of failure the hydraulic fluid trapped by a valve would prevent that happening.

Anyway, even if the slats did retract, the ample power available from the engines would immediately give them sufficient speed to both avoid a stall and have controllability via the ailerons.

The possibility of an engine failure, coupled with an undesired slat retraction, was considered improbable.

However, in the case in question the separation of the engine and pylon damaged the hydraulic lines and caused the slats to retract. Some maintain McDonnell Douglas was taking risks by having so many vulnerable lines just behind the leading edge of the wings.

DC-10 Maintenance and Forewarnings

Reviews of eyewitness reports and examination of the wreckage indicated that the pylon's rear bulkhead flange had been cracked beforehand. In view of the considerable safety margin built in, this could hardly have happened during normal operations and must have happened during maintenance. Indeed, the pylon (together with the engine) had been removed and replaced two months earlier to substitute the bearings.

Investigators found deviations in the maintenance work at a number of airlines. For instance, maintenance workers, on finding certain bolts difficult to remove, would do so in a different order from that specified, thereby placing excess stress on others.

The FAA grounded all United States–registered DC-10s subject to a check of the rear flanges in question. Four American Airlines aircraft and two Continental Airlines aircraft had cracks there. Continental had found their cracks in the rear flanges and replaced them. Other airlines had not experienced that problem.

Forklifts

The reason soon became obvious. The two airlines had devised what they thought was a superefficient way to remove the engine and pylon simultaneously, using a forklift, disregarding the McDonnell Douglas maintenance manual, which said they should be removed individually.

The DC-10's engines are cantilevered far in front of the wing, which means a considerable mechanical moment (levering) is imposed if the engine is lifted more than a certain extent, and that can put tremendous stress on the rear flange. In addition, vibrations from the forklift can be transmitted to it. The accident was partly attributed to poor communication between the parties, namely Continental, the FAA, the manufacturer, and the airlines, regarding the earlier problems at Continental.

DC-10 Grounded for Thirty-Eight Days

This dramatic disaster, which unlike the previous one at Paris was not so much the fault of the manufacturer, led to three airworthiness directives and an almost unheard-of thirty-eight-day grounding of the fleet.

The damage to McDonnell Douglas's reputation in the eyes of the public was so great that many orders for the DC-10 were canceled. The company then dropped behind the competition after failing to develop any more radically new airliners and was finally taken over by Boeing.

Finally, Extremely Safe

The modifications and changes in maintenance procedures introduced following this disaster, coupled with those made in the light of earlier ones related to the cargo door blowing out, meant the DC-10 became statistically one of the safest aircraft.

Pilots who subsequently flew it seemed to appreciate its qualities.

No Room for Two Wide-Body Trijets

Boeing occupied the high ground with the 747, and there was only room for one three-engine wide-body airliner one level down. At the time it had to be three engines, as they were not so reliable in those days and there were not the ETOPS rules allowing twin-engine airliners to fly far from an airport they could divert to in the case of an engine failure.

MacDonnell Douglas did cut some corners to be first and in fact easily won the orders battle, since Lockheed's TriStar L1011, a superb plane with many advanced features, was delayed because Rolls-Royce had problems perfecting its ultimately very successful RB-211 engine.

This commercial setback led to Lockheed's withdrawal from the production of civilian airliners.

Worst-ever Single-aircraft Disaster (Japan, 1985)
Decompression—rush of air damaged hydraulics and tail

> A Boeing 747 staggered drunkenly around the sky for half an hour, with passengers writing last words on their boarding passes.
>
> Japan Airlines Flight 123, August 12, 1985

Off-duty flight attendant Yumi Ochiai felt her hair
lift off her neck and a momentary sense
of weightlessness as the staggering 747
began its final downward plunge.
Trapped between seats, and with a broken pelvis,
she was fitfully aware of the sound of young children,
their cries fading as the injuries, shock,
and cold of the night took their toll.
"I'm a boy," said one in vain to embolden himself.

The Boeing 747 SR (short range), a jumbo specially adapted and reinforced to carry as many as 550 passengers on domestic short-haul routes in Japan, was the early-evening shuttle from Tokyo's domestic Haneda airport to Osaka, Japan's second largest city, four hundred kilometers away to the south. The flight was being flown by First Officer Yutaka Sasaki, thirty-nine, an experienced pilot training for promotion to captain. In the right-hand seat, acting as copilot, was Captain Masami Takahama, forty-nine, a JAL instructor with more than 12,400 hours' experience. Hiroshi Fukuda was the flight engineer.

Unusually, the occupants were mostly women and children, for it was the Obon August holiday period, when the Japanese go back to their hometowns to visit family graves and see relations. The aircraft was virtually full, and most of the passengers were clad in only the lightest of clothes in anticipation of a clammy midsummer evening. As in a number of flights that have ended in disaster, the flight number, JL123, is easy to remember.

Haneda, situated at the edge of Tokyo Bay and very close to the center of the city, had served as Tokyo's international airport until the construction of Narita Airport in the face of fierce opposition some fifty miles (eighty kilometers) away. With little need for noise abatement over the sea, JL123's climb out of Haneda was a simple affair. Ten or so minutes after takeoff, the busy pilots were able to relax. Everything seemed normal.

The first indication the Tokyo controller had that everything was not so came without any forewarning at 7:25 p.m., thirteen minutes after takeoff, and just as JL123 was leveling out at its cruising altitude, when the echo for the aircraft on his radar screen switched to 7700, the emergency code.

Shortly afterward came the following disjointed call from the aircraft:

> Tokyo. Japan Air 123. Request immediate . . . ah . . . trouble. Request return back to Haneda . . . Descend and maintain Flight Level 220.

JL123 then asked for the vector (course) back to Oshima Island, the waypoint on the easiest route over the sea back to Haneda.

The controller gave the crew permission to descend and indicated the appropriate course, but instead of turning 177 degrees to go back on its tracks, JL123 merely made a very slow right turn of some 40 degrees. Surprised by this noncompliance, the Tokyo controller repeated his instructions.

JL123 still did not comply, and with the aircraft heading for dangerous mountains, Japan Airlines' operations center called them on the company frequency, without extracting more information, except that the crew thought a rear cabin door (R5) was broken and that they were going to descend. Watched by the air traffic controllers in Tokyo, the 747 meandered in an area of treacherous mountains not far from Japan's famous Mount Fuji. The pilots kept repeating they were *out of control* while at the same time requesting directions back to Haneda. Periodically losing considerable height and partially regaining it, the aircraft at one point made a tight 360-degree turn.

Finally, after some thirty minutes the echo on the screens showed JL123 rapidly losing altitude, before sinking out of radar view. The controllers vainly hoped the 747 had merely gone into a valley, but getting no reply on the radio, they finally accepted that it must have crashed.

A US transport aircraft taking off from the US Air Force Yokota airbase thirty-five miles away reported seeing fire in the midst of the mountains "that was very likely to be the crashed aircraft."

Who saw what and when is uncertain.

The author read a report that five minutes after the crash the Japanese Air Self-Defense Force had scrambled two F4 Phantom fighters to investigate, and that twenty minutes later they were able to report the presence of fires and the general location as *"299 degrees and 35.5 miles from Yokota US* airbase's TACAN." [A more accurate military beacon]

Certainly, Yokota airbase, in the outer west-northwest suburbs of Tokyo, was relatively near, and it has been said, perhaps in connection with the excellent TV series *Air Crash Investigation*, that a helicopter from Yokota reached the site twenty minutes after the crash but was called back so that the Japanese Self-Defense Forces could take over. (The US military has a privileged but extremely sensitive presence in Japan and scrupulously avoids making any comments that could in any way cause friction, and so it is not easy to check these things out.)

Macarthur Job's *Air Disaster*: Vol. 2 also mentions a Japanese helicopter reaching the site and reporting the wreckage was scattered on a forty-five-degree slope, with fires and virtually no likelihood of any survivors, and that in view of the darkness, rain, and steepness of the terrain, landing there would be impossible. Subsequently, other helicopter crews, working from maps, gave many erroneous locations.

In such terrain, without GPS and with one peak looking very much like another, one had to know the area and have reasonable visibility to get the location right.

Also, it was becoming pitch dark.

Officials, by their very nature, were wondering whether the crash had occurred in Gunma Prefecture or Nagano Prefecture. Which police force would be responsible?

At the time Japan did not have a civil emergency unit to deal with such events. Also, lingering antagonism between the police and fire departments (which at one time had been a single organization) meant, according to some, that the police did not immediately call in the more suitable fire department helicopters. Furthermore, use was not made of US forces, with their considerable experience of plucking downed pilots at night from the mountains of Vietnam, perhaps because of face or the fact that no one wanted to take the responsibility if things went wrong. While in hospital Yumi Ochiai also mentioned hearing helicopter rotors and seeing lights, which could have been those of the US helicopter ordered back or those of the first Japanese helicopter.

In addition, one must remember no one was expecting there to be survivors. Perhaps we are wiser nowadays, with experience showing that at least some of those on board can survive the most horrendous crashes. Adding to the confusion was the absence of high officials, away on the Obon national holiday, the holiday those passengers had been looking forward to enjoying.

To complicate matters, the crash site was in a particularly inaccessible place. No roads came anywhere near, and it was dark. Finally, at 05:37 the *following* morning a Nagano Prefecture police helicopter reported the fuselage was scattered in an area some seven hundred meters east of the prefectural frontier and was all in Gunma Prefecture.

With the site pinpointed, the main rescue teams could set off on what they expected would be a body recovery rather than rescue mission. The earlier reports regarding the fires and the sighting of wreckage scattered over a wide area implied there was little chance anyone could have survived.

Because of the steep tree-covered slopes at the crash site, the authorities had determined that helicopters could not land close to the site even in daylight. To make matters worse, the weather then closed in.

At 08:49, the process of lowering seventy-three paratroopers by rope from giant helicopters hovering over the site began. They were to be the first people on the scene, nearly *fourteen hours* after the crash.

Just as the first paratroopers to descend were confirming by radio at 09:25 that there were no signs of survivors, two members of the Nagano Prefecture rescue team descended at a point one and half miles (2.3 kilometers) away. Subsequently, at 10:15 the neighboring Gunma Prefecture police team arrived on foot, having scaled the mountains.

Four Survivors

Twelve-Year-Old Schoolgirl Symbolizes Disaster

At 10:54, and almost sixteen hours after the crash, a firefighter from Ueno Village and a member of the Nagano Prefecture police rescue team unexpectedly found a survivor trapped in the broken-off part of the rear cabin that had slid some way down the ridge from the main crash area. She was the off-duty JAL flight attendant who heard the cries of the dying children. Next, they found a mother and her eight-year-old daughter under nearby wreckage. All had fractures.

Most surprising of all was the discovery of twelve-year-old Keiko Kawakami in the wreckage of the tail section, with hardly an injury other than a slightly injured arm. Reports that rescuers found her wedged in a tree may be mistaken, as there is a photo of that wreckage with arrows showing the spots where she and the other three of the four survivors were found.

Also, she said she found herself in the wreckage with her mother dead and her father saying he could not help, as he could not move. When he died, she consoled her sister, who was to die too, saying their grandmother would look after them.

A photo taken from the ground showing Keiko being clasped around the waist by a paratrooper in combat gear as the two of them are being winched up into a giant helicopter came to symbolize the disaster. For years, weekly magazines used this eye-catching image to advertise their latest issue with purported new facts about the crash, or failing that, anything showing Japan Airlines in a bad light.

Hopes of further survivors engendered by this good news soon evaporated. Others had survived the impact, and some certainly could have been saved had help come earlier.

What had really happened to the passengers in those thirty minutes leading to the final plunge onto the mountain ridge? What was behind what to this day remains the worst-ever crash involving a single aircraft?

Situation in the Cabin

The flight data recorder and descriptions by the rescued off-duty flight attendant, Yumi Ochiai, reveal how terrifying the thirty-minute roller-coaster ordeal preceding the crash must have been. The aircraft would yaw, pitch, and roll, with each cycle taking about a minute and a half. In addition, there would be the vacillating scream of the engines as the pilots tried to steady the aircraft vertically and horizontally and attempted to nudge it in the direction they wanted. A number of the adults scribbled last words to loved ones on the back of their boarding passes or other scraps of paper.

Situation in the Cockpit

Thanks to the cockpit voice recorder (CVR), the situation in the cockpit is well known, as there are both the crew's conversations between themselves and their exchanges with the air traffic controller—a couple of times the captain tells his colleagues to ignore the air traffic controller and concentrate on keeping the aircraft in the air rather than on ATC.

Although the pilots are speaking in Japanese, there are easily identifiable words from the captain, such as *"Flap up! ... Power! .... Power!"*

Finally, at the end of the half hour, one clearly hears the verbal warnings from the aircraft's ground proximity warning system (GPWS) making a whooping sound, immediately followed by the words *"Pull up!"* repeated five times over a period of nine seconds.

Perhaps the most distressing part is that there follows the sound of one impact, followed a second later by another, as the aircraft sliced a swathe through trees on top of one ridge and plunged down onto another. Then silence.

For the crew it had been a desperate struggle, as the only way they could maneuver the aircraft appeared to be by varying the relative thrust of the engines. At one point they made, as mentioned, a tight 360-degree turn.

Tokyo ATC was calling them, and the nearer American Yokota Air Base was doing likewise. Though the Tokyo controller had suggested Nagoya Airport to the south, they seemed intent on going back to Haneda. Perhaps they were more familiar with it, perhaps because it was "home," and perhaps because it was at the sea's edge and they could ditch the aircraft in the water if their approach failed and they did not come a cropper on the unforgiving sea wall on its perimeter.

The crew knew they had no hydraulic pressure to control the aircraft's control surfaces but did not know why. This in itself was surprising to them, as aircraft manufacturers design these key hydraulic systems with built-in redundancy on the belt-and-braces principle, in that if one fails, one of the others will take over. The systems were in triplicate.

In addition, the crew did not know why the aircraft was so unstable. It was yawing (veering violently from side to side), rolling (one wing tipping down one moment, the other wing the next), and pitching (nose down one moment, nose up the next). Indeed, it was misbehaving in all three axes with a phugoid motion. This porpoise-like pitching, and to some extent the rolling, could be explained by the lack of hydraulics to control the ailerons and elevators, but why was the yawing so considerable? Little did the crew realize that most of the tail plane had been lost.

However, in trying to go back to Haneda instead of going to Nagoya, where they could at least have ditched in the sea en route should they not be able to reach it, they ended up going over the mountainous terrain near Mount Fuji.

When, over the mountains, they repeatedly tried to turn toward Haneda, the aircraft seemed to want to go the other way. Finally, when the speed dropped sufficiently, the first engineer (perhaps on his own initiative) lowered the landing gear. This had the effect of stabilizing the aircraft somewhat but had the disadvantage of making the aircraft lose height and at the same time made it more difficult to steer away from the mountains. The pilots tried lowering the flaps, but this made things worse, so they retracted them just before the crash. (They were able to lower the landing gear and maneuver the flaps by using a backup electrical system.)

They probably were doomed from the moment the incident started thirty minutes earlier. Knowing what we now know, one can say that it was a great feat of airmanship even to stay aloft for so long. In addition, Japan is not a good country in which to be in such a predicament, for it consists mostly of steep volcanic mountains. What little flat ground exists is put to use.

Had the aircraft managed to escape from the high peaks near Mount Fuji to make its way directly to Haneda, it could have crashed in built-up areas, with even greater loss of life. Housing in Japan is often frail and closely packed and the aircraft could have cut a long swath through suburban housing.

The Investigation

No one could understand what had happened, and rumors were rife, and some continue to be so. Had it been hit by a missile? On the other hand, was it a bomb? Was it a meteorite?

Then some solid information began to come in. People on the ground had seen the 747 staggering through the evening sky, and an amateur photographer even had a blurry photo of it *without its vertical tail fin*. A Japanese naval vessel then recovered a large portion of the tail from the sea in the area where the pilot had first declared the emergency some thirty minutes before the crash. Subsequently, searchers recovered other pieces in that area.

Never had there been a structural failure like this on a Boeing 747. The aircraft was relatively old, but there were 747s twice as old still flying safely.

However, as Japan Airlines employed the aircraft on short domestic routes, with many takeoffs and landings, it did have a large number of flight cycles, and it was thought likely that the accident might be linked to that.

A flight cycle is one takeoff and landing and is significant because each time an aircraft climbs into the sky, the pressurized air in the cabin makes the fuselage stretch a little, so everything moves and warps slightly. When the aircraft descends, the opposite happens. Metals do not like constant flexing beyond a certain elastic limit. A phenomenon called "fatigue failure" occurs, where the metal becomes brittle and fails. Anyone who has tried to break a thick copper wire has experienced the phenomenon: one bends it one way and then the opposite several times and it suddenly becomes brittle and breaks.

After the world's first passenger jet (Comet) disasters due to metal fatigue in the late 1950s, manufacturers were very careful to avoid areas of stress concentration. Thus, it was unlikely Boeing had made such a design mistake. Nevertheless, it was very worrying for the company, as the safety of the entire fleet of 747s might be questioned, leading to enormous financial loss. A number of countries immediately ordered their airlines to carry out checks on the tail section.

Boeing sent telexes to all users with information about the maximum number of cycles other 747s had flown without structural trouble. The maximum number of flight cycles for any 747 was 22,970, which was somewhat more than the crashed aircraft's 18,830.

Thus, though JL123's number of cycles was relatively high, it was not deemed excessive.

Investigators began to direct their attention toward the rear pressure bulkhead, which though made of quite thin material is a kind of plug keeping the pressurized air in the cabins from escaping through the rear of the aircraft. However, Boeing had designed it to last at least twenty years and the crashed aircraft was only eleven years old. The bulkhead could have failed because of corrosion—indeed, another type of aircraft flying out of London had crashed due to corrosion of the rear pressure bulkhead fourteen years previously—but there was no sign of corrosion on the JAL bulkhead.

Then one of Boeing's investigators discovered a small piece of the rear pressure bulkhead with repairs made using a splice and rivets, with merely a single row of rivets. How could there only be a single row of rivets when Boeing, for the very fatigue failure reason mentioned above, always mandated that there be a double row of rivets to prevent concentrated stress leading to fatigue cracking?

Records showed the aircraft had suffered a tail strike seven years earlier on landing at Osaka Airport with its nose too high in the air and had been out of service for three months for repairs. Boeing immediately thought they were off the hook, as it was assumed Japan Airlines had been responsible for the incorrect repairs. Then to their consternation they discovered the repairs had been carried out under the supervision of, and according to instructions from, their own engineers sent over from the States!

There followed a period of buck-passing. Japan Airlines said Boeing was responsible for the crash due to the faulty repairs; Boeing said it was Japan Airlines' fault for not having detected the crack. One of Boeing's arguments was that as the Japanese are chronic smokers, there must have been visible signs of tar on the edges of the developing crack on the far side (from the cabin).

Japan Airlines countered by saying it was in a visually inaccessible place, and anyway, no one would expect to see anything wrong at such a spot in the absence of signs of corrosion, say from water from the toilets or galley. These fatigue cracks can take years to develop and might have been virtually invisible early on.

Allegedly, Japan Airlines accepted 20 percent of the blame on the grounds that for an extended period up to the disaster, whistling had been heard at the back of the aircraft in question and no one had checked it out.

Boeing

Finally, both companies realized their slanging match was mutually damaging and decided to compromise. After all, Japan Airlines was a major Boeing customer, and falling out with it could in the long term cost much more. Another point was that the accident happened in Japan, where there is not the lawyer compensation culture found in the United States, and the payouts were not as great as they might have been.

After arranging for some free modifications to existing 747s worldwide to ensure that failure, however unlikely, of another rear bulkhead would not result in catastrophic consequential damage, Boeing finally came out of the affair relatively unscathed.

Japan Airlines

The same was not true for Japan Airlines. No one could prove it was entirely its fault, but the Japanese press turned on it like a lynch mob. This was partly due to the haughty attitude the featherbedded airline had shown over the years. The media hounded it relentlessly, picking up on every possible fault. It took years for it to recover, and perhaps domestically it never quite has.

In Japan it is always felt that someone should take the blame and demonstrate his or her contrition. In the case of the 747 disaster, the police treated the crash site as a crime scene and only let the investigators borrow the debris. The main purpose of air accident investigations in the West is to determine the cause so a similar thing does not occur again, but even in the United States there is an increasing tendency to obfuscate, since the potential legal liability can be so costly. However, where the impartiality of the accident investigators might later be questioned, as in the case of the Airbus crash at a tiny air show in France, there is something to be said for judicial authorities ensuring flight recorders are not tampered with, assuming the judicial authorities can be trusted.

In the following months, someone at JAL did commit suicide, leading the press to conclude he was the man responsible for the bad repairs or for not finding the crack in the pressure bulkhead.

In fact, the suicide had nothing to do with the crash. Yet if someone at JAL *had* felt personally responsible, that individual might well have committed suicide. For instance, around about that time there was a sad case where passengers who had had omelet for breakfast on a JAL flight staggered off the aircraft at Tokyo with serious food poisoning. A young JAL cook at the Anchorage stopover with an infected hand had handled the mixture of blended eggs, which had presumably been left standing uncooked. No one died, but he committed suicide, nevertheless. Most safety experts would now say it was a systems or management failure, for the airline should have ensured the cook had gloves or had been kept off work—he had been too conscientious, returning to work.

Conclusion

The conclusions were that to prevent such accidents one should:

1. Find ways to avoid and detect such maintenance or repair mistakes through better management (oversight) and improved checks.
2. Ensure one failure does not result in collateral damage that could endanger the aircraft.

The author has heard it suggested that had Japan Airlines carried out maintenance less assiduously and left holes and weak parts in the fuselage behind the bulkhead, the air would have been able to escape through those without blowing off the tail fin!

Was Depressurization Really So Rapid?

A retired JAL pilot, Hideo Fujita, has written a book entitled *Kakusareta Shougen* (Hidden Testimony), in which he doubts that sudden depressurization ever occurred and says that the cause of the accident must lie elsewhere. His reasons for doubting that the decompression was as sudden as claimed are:

1. The pilots were able to continue physically demanding movements without donning their oxygen masks for some time, even though the aircraft was at twenty-one thousand feet, where the air is thin.

2. The rescued off-duty flight attendant, Yumi Ochiai, had heard a bang above her, not behind her, and had seen no papers flying around in any direction, which one would have expected had the air been rushing out of a big hole. (In the author's opinion, the panels of the tail fin could have been blown off without the immediate exodus of a large volume of air.)

3. Shortly after the crash, Japan Airlines said the rescued off-duty flight attendant had said she had seen air coming out of the floor vents, when in fact she could not have seen them from her seat and had never heard of the term.

Whatever the truth, it is certain that the official cause of the crash being faulty repairs by individuals was very convenient for Boeing and even JAL.

Late Arrival of Rescuers

The report from a helicopter arriving early above the crash scene that there were surely no survivors was a factor in rescuers not arriving earlier.

The Americans, who were probably the best placed to help, were kept away. The US military presence in Japan is such a delicate issue that no one on the US side would want to comment. However, judging by the appreciation shown for the help given by the US forces in connection with the 2011 earthquake and tsunami, attitudes may have changed radically.

The slopes were too steep and tree covered for helicopters to land even in daylight, and potential survivors would have been in the tail section, which had broken off and slipped down the steep slope, ending up quite some distance from the main site. They would have been difficult to find in the dark, notwithstanding the cries and moans mentioned by Yumi Ochiai.

Respect for the Dead

Another footnote to the JL123 disaster is that for the Japanese families, as in any disaster involving Japanese, the proper handling and fullest possible recovery of the bodies and all their parts were of the utmost importance. Senior people from the airline attended every funeral, and staff visit the crash site on every anniversary.

737 Rudder Quirk Took Years to Demonstrate (1991/1994)
Two disasters and almost a third

> A story of the investigation as much as of the incidents.
>
> FDRs at the time did not reveal how the pilots actuated the controls, so they were easily suspect.
>
> United Airlines Flight 585, March 3, 1991
> USAir Flight 427, September 8, 1994
> Eastwind Airlines Flight 517, June 9, 1996

The First Incident at Colorado Springs:
United Airlines Flight 585

With no warning, the United Airlines Boeing 737 from Denver rolled sharply to the right as it approached Colorado Springs Airport. Then the nose pitched down. Abandoning the landing, the pilots increased thrust and reset the flaps to fifteen degrees to recover. But on down they went, in a tight spiral, sustaining accelerations over 4 g before crashing in a park less than four miles from the runway, killing all the occupants.

Mercifully, there had been only twenty-five people on board, and this is why the accident did not receive the attention it might have.

With their usual due diligence, the NTSB investigated the crash but, unusually, were unable to determine the cause, partly because at the time and for some time afterward cockpit data recorders were very primitive. In this Colorado crash only five parameters were recorded, namely heading, altitude, airspeed, g loads (vertical acceleration), and microphone keying. All parameters were sampled and recorded once per second, except vertical acceleration, which was sampled eight times per second.

In fact, it was not the recorder that was primitive but the aircraft, in that unlike today's airliners it was controlled by wire cables that physically pulled actuators, with no need for sensors that could provide data to the recorder capable of handling many more parameters.

The fragmentation of the aircraft and damage by fire made finding informative physical evidence difficult. The rudder power control unit (PCU), which was a key item, was too damaged for valid testing. Nevertheless, there were the radar tracks and reports from hundreds of witnesses.

What made this investigation, and the one for a similar crash three and a half years later, so inconclusive was there was no means to tell exactly what the pilots did, such as did they crazily stomp on the rudder pedal, and if they did, which one?

There were two main theories as to its likely cause:

1. The power control unit (PCU) caused a rudder "hardover," making the aircraft veer to the right and tip downward at the low speed it was flying at in preparation for landing.

2. Strong vortices of swirling air (mountain rotors), known to have been present in that general area but not necessarily at that location, had upset the aircraft.

Boeing considered the latter more likely, with the pilots very likely having stupidly stomped on one of the rudder pedals. However, a study of the fifty-two-year-old captain's and forty-two-year-old first officer's backgrounds suggested that neither he nor she would ever have done such a thing.

One should explain that rudders, unlike those on ships, are not much used on airliners. To turn, the pilot, human or automatic, uses the ailerons to bank the aircraft to the side toward which they want to go, after which the aircraft turns naturally. Otherwise, the rudder is mainly only used when landing in a crosswind.

The reason why airliners, such as the 737, with the engines attached way out to the wings rather than close in to the fuselage have such enormous rudders is to correct the tremendous torque produced when an engine fails and they should be able to fly (safely) on one engine pulling just on one side.

For simplicity, slim design, and cheap maintenance, the 737 was virtually unique in having what, on the one hand, was a very simple rudder system but, on the other, depended on a too-clever-by-half, two-in-one rudder power control unit. This control unit was designed by Boeing's engineers and manufactured for them by the Parker Hannifin Corporation per their specifications.

Other airliners had three PCUs and even split rudders so that if one half did an unwarranted hardover, the other half could easily compensate, with the effect anyway half what it otherwise would be. The 737 had a standby PCU that could be activated by the pilots if necessary, and *if* they had time.

Though Boeing considered a rudder hardover most unlikely on the 737, they claimed it could be handled, provided the pilots dealt with it correctly. However, this depended on their knowing what to do and the airspeed being high enough for the ailerons to be able to compensate.

The Second Incident, at Hopewell: USAir Flight 427

Tom Haueter, a senior investigator at the NTSB, was on call, having offered to stand in as a favor for a colleague wanting to go on holiday. Little did he know that would mean being bestowed with an investigation that was to dominate part of his life and even strain his marriage due to the unrelenting calls on his time, day and night, for months and months.

That day he was head of the go-team, consisting of experts in various domains always ready to go to any air crash at a moment's notice. They were in Washington, DC, and the crash had been at Hopewell Township, about nine miles from Pittsburgh International Airport, and almost an hour's flying time from where they were.

The first problem Haueter faced was mundane but not simple: finding a hotel they could use as a base for the investigations and a place for the team to stay and liaise. USAir had booked them all, and it was only after much effort that Haueter managed to persuade the airline to give one up—the Holiday Inn near Pittsburgh Airport.

It was late in the evening, and the pilots of the FAA aircraft they would be using had run out of hours. They would have to fly down to Pittsburgh the following morning.

When Haueter did finally reach the USAir Flight 427 crash site, he found body parts everywhere—even hanging from trees. He declared the site a biohazard, meaning his staff would have to wear full-body biohazard suits for their protection as they fumbled through the wreckage looking for evidence, which had to be disinfected before being taken away for further study.

All 132 occupants—127 passengers and 5 crew—on board the Boeing 737-300 had died on impact.

For simplicity, we shall refer to this second 737 crash, which had much in common with the Colorado one, as the Hopewell crash.

USAir Flight 427, a Boeing 737-300, had departed from Chicago for Palm Beach, Florida, with a stopover at Pittsburgh.

As it approached Pittsburgh International Airport, it encountered the wake of Delta Flight 1083, a Boeing 727-200, about to land before them. The 727 was four miles ahead, and vortices produced would not in theory have been enough to engender a sustained changing of heading without input from the pilots.

The aircraft yawed slightly to the left, banked to the left, and rolled over twice leftward before hitting the ground upside down in a wooded area with a dirt road.

At first it seemed to Haueter and his colleagues that the investigation might be over more quickly than usual. The cockpit data recorder showed the aircraft had yawed and rolled to the left; this and other evidence clearly pointed to a rudder malfunction and, unlike in the first incident, the suspect power control unit (PCU) controlling the rudder had been recovered fully intact.

In fact, it was to take more than four and a half years before the NTSB would be able to draw the investigation to a satisfactory conclusion, and this process was greatly helped and given traction by a further incident, which fortunately resulted in no fatalities.

The Third Incident: Eastwind Airlines Flight 517

An Eastwind Airlines Boeing 737-201 reported a loss of rudder control while on approach to Richmond, Virginia. The airplane was on a regularly scheduled passenger flight from Trenton, NJ to Richmond, with forty-eight passengers, two pilots, and three flight attendants on board. Apart from a minor injury to a flight attendant, there were no injuries or damage to the airplane as a result of the incident.

At the time of the event, the aircraft's airspeed was about 250 knots, and it was at four thousand feet MSL.

The captain reported that he was hand flying the airplane and he felt a slight rudder bump to the right. As he was asking the first officer whether he had felt the bump, the aircraft suddenly rolled to the right. He applied opposite rudder but said he felt the rudder resist.

He said he then applied opposite aileron and used asymmetric power to keep the airplane upright. He stated that after he declared an emergency to the approach controller, he and the first officer performed the emergency checklist. The captain reported that as part of the checklist they turned off the yaw damper. He reported that the airplane became controllable but was not certain as to whether the problem went away at the same time as the yaw damper was turned off. The aircraft rolled over again but that time to the right. After another thirty seconds, the plane snapped back to level flight.

It is reported that the airplane has previously had problems with uncommanded rudder deflections. Previous reports had been of "rudder bumps" during departure and that the airplane would not trim properly. The FDR was removed from the airplane for examination.

The next day, people from the NTSB bombarded the pilots with probing questions. Here, at last, they had the aircraft and the pilots intact.

The Investigation(s)

The Colorado investigation had got nowhere, and after three and a half years the NTSB had officially admitted they could not determine probable cause—only one of four instances where that had been the case.

Still present were some of the factors that had made that investigation so difficult in the Hopewell disaster, one of which was that the cockpit data recorder, although providing slightly more information, did not record what the pilots did with the rudder pedals. This gave Boeing much wiggle room, with them able to claim (and to some extent believe) the pilots again stomped on the pedals mistakenly on being startled by the wake turbulence from the 727 ahead.

The NTSB investigators had faced a conundrum in that the Boeing 737 was too safe. Three and a half years had elapsed between the Colorado and Hopewell disasters, with the first having few fatalities, and so many 737s were flying safely worldwide. Even recommending a different rudder system would be very expensive, and anyway, the lengthy approval system meant that it would take time to come into effect, especially if it were ordered without convincing proof of its necessity.

To be fair, Boeing had not stinted on getting hundreds of engineers and experts to consider the matter and genuinely thought reasons other than the PCU were probably responsible. If they had definite proof, they would have acted, notably at the instigation of their lawyers, as they did later.

With even some at the NTSB having doubts after years of theorizing, tests, and meetings, the Eastwind incident was a shot in the arm for Haueter and the NTSB investigators, not only because it provided more material, but also because it gave credence to their belief that it was not the pilots but the PCU that must have been at fault.

Two similar cases might be coincidence, but three would be beyond coincidence.

This knowledge helped sustain Haueter in his endeavor to find proof, and that proof came from dogged determination to pursue the search, though almost by chance. The revelation came in two parts.

Firstly, with the NTSB having been clutching at straws for so long, Jim Hall, chairman of the NTSB, who was a politician rather than a man with technical expertise himself, decided that a panel of the best experts in the domain of hydraulics and associated valves should review what had been done. Collaborating with the panel was a team under the NTSB's Greg Phillips, responsible for systems evaluation.

When the panel met, one of its members, sixty-seven-year-old Ralph Vick, mentioned to Phillips how thirty years before, while working at Bendix on a valve in the hope of a contract from Boeing for the 747, they had done a thermal shock test and found the valve jammed; however, when redesigned with different tolerances, it didn't. Could they try that?

Out of ideas, they did, albeit under somewhat primitive conditions, and found the new valve from the factory never jammed but the one from the crash did. What is more, when taken apart and examined by Hannifin Parker, the precision parts showed no marks indicating any jamming.

This was not quite the Eureka moment it was reported to have been in some accounts, for while showing it could jam without leaving any evidence, it did not explain the hardover. Furthermore, as Boeing insisted, the extreme conditions under which the thermal shock test had been carried out were impossible in the conditions under which the 737 flew.

Secondly, six weeks later, Phillips' team went to a Boeing laboratory in Seattle to run the test under more sophisticated conditions with better monitoring. Again, the factory unit passed, while the one from the crash failed the most extreme thermal shock test. The technician moving the valve back and forth felt it slow down; he didn't notice it bind, but a computer showed it had jammed momentarily. He repeated the action and felt the lever kick back when he tried to move it to the right. When he tried again, he felt it stick to the left and then jam.

In his excellent book *The Mystery of Flight 427: Inside a Crash Investigation*, which took six years to research and write, Bill Adair explains what happened next.

> "Despite their skepticism, Boeing engineers said they would examine the charts from the tests for anything unusual. A few days later, in a building overlooking Paine Field in Everett, a young Boeing engineer named Ed Kikta sat at his desk, reviewing the charts. He could see the test data on his computer screen, but he liked to print the results so he could study them more closely. The charts showed the flow of hydraulic fluid during each test: higher when it was pushing the rudder and down to zero when it was not. Kikta expected that when the outer valve jammed during the thermal shock, the inner valve would compensate and send an equal amount of fluid in the opposite direction,

which would keep the rudder at neutral. That was the great safety feature of the 737 valve. It could compensate for a jam.

But as Kikta studied the squiggly lines for the return flow, he saw dips that were not supposed to be there. When he matched them to another graph showing the force on the levers inside the PCU, he made an alarming discovery. When the outer valve had jammed, the inner valve had moved too far to compensate. That meant the rudder would not have returned to neutral, the way it was supposed to.

The rudder would have reversed. That could be catastrophic. A pilot would push on the left pedal, expecting the rudder to go left, but it would go right."

That was the real Eureka moment.

Kikta's colleagues and boss confirmed the significance of his findings, and Boeing ordered the PCU manufacturer, Parker Hannifin, to check out the results. Their engineers confirmed them, adding that the levers in the PCU could flex, allowing the inner valve to line up with the wrong holes!

Boeing wasted no time. Taking a new 737 straight off the production line, they installed a PCU specially made by Parker Hannifin to simulate the jam. With Kikta on a trestle watching the rudder and PCU, they had a Boeing test pilot play around with the rudder pedals.

At first nothing out of the ordinary was found, but when the test pilot pressed on the left pedal and then pressed down as hard as he could on the right one, it kicked back violently. Further tests showed that how the inner slide behaved depended on where the outer one jammed.

Aware how serious the situation was, Boeing went into overdrive, gathering their engineers to seek a solution. The next day they informed the FAA but asked for twenty-four hours to work out what should be done.

The fact that the NTSB was the last to be informed might seem to have been something of a slight. In fact, as the NTSB can only recommend, and it is the FAA that regulates at its discretion, according or not to whatever the NTSB says, it made sense for Boeing to do all they could to keep the FAA on side. Though Haueter had been in a meeting all day in the presence of someone from Boeing, that person never mentioned the latest findings—he later denied he knew. Haueter only found out by text message from his boss the following morning, who himself had just got the news from the FAA.

Boeing sent telexes to all airlines using the 737, warning them that under certain conditions some jams of the secondary slide could result in anomalous rudder motion.

Haueter carried out further tests and concluded that a rudder-induced disaster required an extremely rare combination of circumstances. It concerned just one percent of the PCUs with certain inherent characteristics where the aircraft encountered turbulence to which the pilot reacted in a certain way, and where the airspeed on coming in to land was too low for the ailerons to be able to override the effect of the rudder. (The airspeed above which the ailerons could override the ailerons being called the crossover speed.) By naturally pulling back on the control column in an effort to save themselves, the pilots were only making their predicament worse.

Haueter, with his colleagues' and bosses' support, finally got the NTSB board to make a final determination, thus ending an investigation that had taken five years, or almost ten if one includes the first incident.

However, publicity-wise, Boeing rather took the wind out of the NTSB sails by preempting them, saying they were taking measures to make the 737 *even* safer.

Oddly, unlike the McDonnell Douglas DC-10, where the second crash—largely due to the way the aircraft had been maintained by raising an engine with a forklift, putting too much strain on a component—resulted in the public and airlines losing faith in the aircraft, they never feared to fly on the 737.

We have only been able to touch on aspects of the longest air crash investigation ever. It finally ensured the most widely used airliner would be "even" safer.

Bill Adair's book explains it all in detail, and notably the party system, by which the relatively minuscule NTSB, with only limited resources, allows all parties to be part of its investigations. It thereby gets results it otherwise might not, despite each party fighting its corner until the truth becomes undeniable. No one knows an aircraft or component better than its maker, and nowadays that increasingly includes the software.

However, it does have the drawback that the maker of a component that could have caused a crash for which it could be liable for enormous damages is sent that component for initial evaluation, as in the 737 SilkAir "suicide" disaster described elsewhere in this book.

There would seem to be a case for the NTSB to be better funded and able to fund more independent work.

Boeing redesigned the rudder mechanism, dispensing with the clever two-in-one PCU and replacing it with a dual input PCU and an automatically activated standby PCU. They also incorporated additional safety features, including some recommended by the NTSB. Work on existing 737s was done largely at Boeing's great expense.

There was one further scare, in rather different circumstances, implying the failure mode was even more complicated than that determined, but none after the modifications, apart from issues related to quality control in the manufacture of the control rods.

Northwest 747 Lower Rudder Hardover (Anchorage, 2002)

But, could pilots still control aircraft on slowing to land?

The popular press tends to say a pilot is "fighting at the controls" when they are doing more harm than good. In this case, they were truly, and physically, fighting at the controls, miles far from any airport.

Northwest Airlines Flight 85, October 9, 2002

Being the launch customer for an aircraft has its advantages, including publicity and very keen prices. However, a number of bugs might still have to be worked out, causing expensive delays and canceled departures. Though launch issues cannot be directly linked to what occurred in this instance, the aircraft happened to be the first production Boeing 747-400, delivered to Northwest Airlines on December 8, 1989.

The flight had taken off from Detroit, with 386 passengers and 18 crew, bound for Tokyo's Narita Airport, a flight of thirteen hours or so. Much of the early part had been over the US and Canada and the US again (Alaska).

Unlike the early 747s, which had ninety or more dials and switches to watch over, these later 747s had computers and no need for a flight engineer. However, some of the control surfaces had semi-direct manual control, unlike the latest fly-by-wire airliners, where a signal is sent electronically or otherwise to actuators that do all the work, though some sensation might be simulated to give the pilots the feel they are flying it.

Because of the flight's thirteen-hour duration, there were two flight crews, and as the 747 left Alaska and headed out over the Bering Sea, Senior Captain John Hanson and First Officer David Smith were settling in to relax and rest while Captain Frank Geib and First Officer Mike Fagan did the actual flying up front in the cockpit.

At the halfway point above the Bering Sea Captain Hanson felt the aircraft perform an odd maneuver. He and First Officer Smith immediately began putting on their uniforms, and no sooner had the aircraft recovered than the special chime sounded to indicate their presence was needed in the cockpit right away.

On arriving there, they found Relief Captain Geib literally fighting at the controls. The control wheel was about halfway over—something that would never happen in cruise—and Geib's right leg was straining on the right rudder pedal. Yet the instrument panel showed that the lower rudder was at the left (opposite) stop and, surprisingly, at a deflection of seventeen degrees, when at altitude the aircraft would never allow it to exceed about six degrees. They were at thirty-five thousand feet.

Captain Geib told them that the airplane, on autopilot, had suddenly begun an uncommanded roll to the left that reached almost forty-five degrees before he realized that the autopilot could not cope and disengaged it. By pressing as hard as he could on the right rudder pedal to move the upper rudder to the right and using the ailerons, he just managed to correct the bank. Had he not reacted quickly, the aircraft would have tipped right over and plunged earthward.

With Tokyo more than six hours' flying time away and Anchorage only two, he had made a gentle left turn—the only direction in which he could—back to the latter. Too far from Anchorage, they had to contact another Northwest airliner to ask them to relay their messages to the controllers.

Their manuals had solutions for almost every conceivable problem but said nothing about the one they faced. Later they were able to contact Northwest by flaky HF radio, but they had no suggestions either. Unable to see the tail, they were in constant fear that the situation might deteriorate or that it might even break off, leaving them helpless.

As senior captain, Captain Hanson had taken over from Captain Geib, even though he had done a sterling job. Because of the physical effort needed to keep pressing down on the right rudder pedal, Hanson and copilot First Officer Fagan took turns.

Not knowing how the aircraft would behave when slowed for landing, they decided to approach Anchorage at about fourteen thousand feet, which, according to Hanson, "is a nice intermediate altitude. It's low enough that the air is nice and thick, and it's high enough that if you do lose control you can make one good honest attempt at recovery before the water."

They managed to land safely, even keeping the aircraft straight on the runway, so the feared emergency evacuation proved unnecessary.

Investigation

The fault causing the problem was found to be a most unlikely one, namely fatigue fracture of the lower rudder power control module manifold—a part that should have lasted forever. The module was redesigned with internal stops so that in the unlikely event of a reoccurrence, the deflection of the rudder would be limited and easily handled.

DHL Airbus Maneuvered by Engine Power Alone (Baghdad, 2003)

A feat that did not receive publicity it merited

> Outside Homeland Security circles, not much attention has been paid to this remarkable feat.
>
> The three-man crew of an Airbus A300B4 freighter brought it safely back to Baghdad Airport by juggling engine power alone after it had been struck by a surface-to-air missile (SAM).
>
> DHL Cargo Flight, Baghdad, November 2, 2003

Some superior surface-to-air missiles possessed by insurgents in Iraq had a maximum range of four and half kilometers at heights up to about ten thousand feet.

Aircraft coming into Baghdad would keep well above that ceiling and descend spirally at the last minute with degrees of bank impossible to practice in simulators set with the conventional parameters. However, departure from Baghdad was riskier for workhorse aircraft—as opposed to fighters—unable to climb quickly.

As a result, the DHL Airbus freighter that took off from Baghdad at midmorning on November 22, 2003 was only climbing through eight thousand feet at 9:15 a.m. when one of the two Russian-made SAM-14s fired from the ground struck it near the left wingtip.

The crew, consisting of two Belgians, Captain Eric Gennotte and First Officer Steeve Michielsen, and Scottish flight engineer Mario Rofail, felt a judder, followed shortly by an alarm indicating trouble with the hydraulics.

The flight engineer saw that two of the three independent systems showed zero pressure and a complete loss of fluid.

Before the crew could go through the steps required for flying with just one hydraulic system operable, the pressure in the third and only remaining system dropped to zero. The instruments also seemed to indicate the fuel in the outboard left-wing fuel tank had disappeared.

Like in the cases of the "uncontrollable" JAL 747 and the Sioux City DC-10, their only hope lay in varying the engine thrust to direct the aircraft, except that compared to the JAL 747, they still had the complete vertical stabilizer (tail fin) to steady them—but not steer them—horizontally. Even so, the aircraft yawed to the left and the left wing began to sink, with the nose dropping. However, by adjusting the relative thrusts of the engines—more power on the left, less on the right—it was possible to correct this before the craft entered into a sideslip and spin, from which it would have been impossible to recover without the help of the rudder and ailerons driven by hydraulic power.

On limping back toward the airport, they were erroneously informed by the tower that the left engine was on fire. From their position on the flight deck, and with no cabin crew (and no windows, since it was a freighter), the crew were unable to see the extensive damage to the left wing.

They had some measure of control, but, concerned about the alleged engine fire, they did not dare spend time experimenting, like the pilots of the Sioux City DC-10 had been able to do.

They were intent on landing but found they were too high and going too fast to risk it without the use of air brakes and abort it.

This meant they had to make a time-consuming circuit getting far enough out to be able to make a shallow approach that they could manage. The pilot of a US Apache helicopter had informed them that it was not the engine that was on fire but the wing extremity. This was somewhat reassuring, but with fuel leaking from the wing there was the danger that fuel for that engine would run out. With no power pushing it up, that wing would tip downward, and they would plunge to the ground.

The only plus was that, having lowered the undercarriage for the landing, the aircraft after a few scary moments had become slightly easier to control.

On their second attempt, some sixteen minutes after the missile strike, they were aiming for Runway 33R but fortunately had veered to the left one and, caught up by turbulence at about 400 feet (120 meters), had to increase thrust to raise the right wing, touching down just off the centerline of 33L, the runway parallel to it on the left. "Touched" down is something of a misnomer, as they came down hard with a sink rate of some two thousand feet a minute instead of the usual maximum of three hundred feet a minute, and an airspeed of roughly 215 knots instead of the usual 140 knots or so.

Rofail immediately deployed full reverse thrust, but the Airbus veered off the paved runway to the left—had they been on the right-hand runway, they would have hit the fire station.

The aircraft ran through rough soft ground, throwing up a plume of sand and dragging a razor-wire barrier, coming to a halt in about 3,300 feet (1,000 meters). With no hydraulics to operate the steering, they were unable to correct their course.

With no brakes, no spoilers, and no flaps, they only had reverse thrust to slow the fast-moving aircraft. Once off the runway, a 600-meter run through the sand with sparse grass helped bring the hurtling aircraft to a halt at a razor-wire barrier. The crew were able to evacuate safely down a second chute after finding the first damaged by the razor wire.

With emergency vehicles rushing to the scene at the airport perimeter, the three men who evacuated via that emergency slide, were stunned they had survived. Standing on the hot sand, they were about to make their way to the emergency vehicles, which, surprisingly, had held back.

"Don't move!" someone shouted. "You are in a dangerous zone with unexploded ordinance."

One of the drivers said he would back up to them—if the rear wheels did set anything off it would be far away from the cab—and drive out with them following in his tire tracks, which they duly did.

The nightmare was over.

Backstory

On that day, Claudine Vernier, a journalist for Paris Match magazine, who had been interviewing insurgents, was invited out with her cameraman to see them in action. Taken to an area near the airport, she was surprised to see masked men carrying missile launchers. The leader explained the difference between the SAM-14 and SAM-7, after which they made ready to fire a SAM-14 at an aircraft that had just taken off, in fact the DHL A300. Only then did the two journalists realize the insurgents were not bluffing.

Seeing they had hit the aircraft but that it was still flying, the insurgents fired a second missile, a less effective SAM-7, which missed.

Afterwards, the journalists were criticized for not having interceded, but Vernier said that would not have made any difference, except perhaps getting them shot in the head. They realized they had been set up. Their videos can be found on the Internet and were used in the *MAYDAY/Air Crash Investigations* portrayal.

Technical Points—Damage to Aircraft

The missile struck the rear tip of the left wing, setting the fuel tank on fire, but did not cause it to explode as, being full of fuel just after takeoff, there was no vapor. The slipstream meant the leaking fuel was burning along the trailing edge of the wing, with it being gradually eaten away, reaching the main spar, which was on the point of failing when they touched down.

A large section of the left wing was missing when they landed, making one wonder how it provided the lift that it did.

Aftermath—Airliners at Risk Almost Everywhere

The three-man aircrew were officially honored for their great achievement, which, with no passengers involved and not in full view in a major city, did not receive the publicity it deserved.

The crew, consisting of two Belgians—thirty-eight-year-old Captain Éric Gennotte and twenty-nine-year-old First Officer Steeve Michielsen—and a Scot, fifty-four-year-old Flight Engineer Mario Rofail, claimed they owed their success largely to how well they worked together as a team.

This highlights the fact that the "extra pair of hands"— in this case the presence of Flight Engineer Mario Rofail, and in the Sioux City miracle landing (see Chapter 10) the presence of off-duty company DC-10 check and training captain Dennis Fitch, who, too, helped manipulate the controls—made all the difference.

Rofail said in an interview with the UK's *Flight International*, "Situations like this are unique every time. You cannot train for them."

However, some think you can and looked into ways pilots might be trained to cope. Not only that, it has been suggested that aircraft computers could be programmed so that pilots can switch to "thrust control," letting the autopilot fly the aircraft according to what the pilots input into the flight management system without them touching the controls.

The trouble is that total failure of the hydraulic systems is so rare it is not deemed worth the expenditure. Interestingly, when an engine of a Qantas A380 superjumbo disintegrated after the aircraft took off from Singapore, damaging many of the hydraulic systems, the fact that a number of functions were powered electrically rather than hydraulically helped make the incident survivable.

Another thing not deemed worth the expenditure for civilian operations, except for special cases, such as El Al and other Israeli airlines, the US president's Air Force Ones, and aircraft used by other notables, is having antimissile defenses incorporated in the aircraft.

These normally depend on detecting the missile and deploying chaff and flares to confuse it, or firing lasers to interfere with it. However, that is often not enough, for the pilots have to be trained to take avoiding action as well.

Israeli airlines found some countries unhappy with the fact that their flares might accidentally start fires.

While such measures can defeat heat-seeking MANPADS, such as those used against the DHL A300 at Baghdad, they would not be effective against radar-locking missiles, such as the BUK surface-to-air missile that shot down Malaysian Airlines Flight MH17 over Ukraine.

At the moment, the only option is to avoid conflict zones and rely on intelligence to foil plots elsewhere, which could be anywhere.

The crew were showered with praise and received awards in recognition of their great feat of airmanship. Flight Engineer Mario Rofail retired, but the other two continued flying.

DHL resumed service to Baghdad a week later, carrying letters and other items for the troops

Chapter 7
FIRE AND SMOKE

Fire in Varig 707 Toilet on Approach to Orly (Paris, 1973)

Blinded by dense smoke in cockpit, pilots land short

> With the high cost of aircraft, and passengers' and crews' lives so valuable, it is surprising that smoke detectors in the toilets were not in use at the time of this accident. Unbelievably, they were only made mandatory in the United States after an in-flight fire in a washroom ten years later.
>
> Varig Flight 820, July 11, 1973

Friends and relatives of passengers on the Brazilian Varig flight from Rio de Janeiro about to land at Paris's Orly Airport were impatiently watching the arrivals board. They could not understand the delay, as it was well past the expected time still being indicated on the board.

These were old-style mechanical boards, where the letters and numbers flip over until they arrive at the right one. They flipped again, mystifying those waiting.

For instead of "Landed" being next to their flight number, there were the troubling words "Contact Company."

This was somewhat different from what happened when an Air France A330 on the same route from Rio de Janeiro plunged into the South Atlantic in 2009.

Even though the airline knew the aircraft had been lost many hours before its scheduled arrival in Paris, the signboards used the much kinder term "Delayed."

At Orly in 1973, surprise changed to alarm as the assembled greeters began to grasp that something terribly wrong must have happened. Only later did they learn that a fire had broken out in one of the aircraft's aft toilets not far from them on the final approach to the airport, not far from where they were.

Informed by the pilots of the onboard fire, air traffic control (ATC) had duly authorized the captain of Varig Flight 820, Gilberto Araujo da Silva, to make a quick straight-in landing. Despite being able to breathe, thanks to their full-face oxygen masks, the pilots opted to crash-land five kilometers short of the runway, as the smoke was so dense they could not even see their instruments and had to stick their heads out of the cockpit windows to see where they were going.

Ten occupants—all crew members—managed to escape. Fire crews, arriving some six to seven minutes later, were only able to rescue four unconscious people, just one of whom subsequently survived.

In all, 7 crew and 116 passengers died.

Most of the deaths were by inhalation of carbon monoxide and other toxic products resulting from the fire. For some passengers, it would have been like a prison gas chamber, since hydrogen cyanide was one of the gases given off by the smoldering plastics.

This accident led to the overdue installation of smoke detectors in some aircraft toilets, a review of air supply to flight decks, and a review of the plastics used in cabin interiors.

Surprisingly, it was not this event, outside the United States, that made the FAA mandate that aircraft lavatories be equipped with smoke detectors and automatic fire extinguishers, but the 1983 Cincinnati Air Canada Flight 797 in-flight fire in the United States ten years later! The FAA mandated that within five years jetliners be retrofitted with fire-blocking layers on seat cushions and floor lighting to lead passengers to exits in dense smoke.

In the case of Air Canada 797, the DC-9 was flying at thirty-three thousand feet from Dallas to Toronto when a fire developed in the area of a rear toilet. Before long the cabin began to fill with thick black smoke as the aircraft made an emergency descent. As in the Varig case just described, the smoke was so dense the pilots had difficulty seeing their instruments. In their case they did manage to land at Cincinnati Airport, but shortly after the doors and emergency exits had been opened, a flash fire swept through the cabin before everyone had had time to escape, with the result that half of the forty-six people on board died.

Possibly the Varig incident awakened the authorities to the obvious need for fire detectors in aircraft toilets, while the Cincinnati incident confirmed it.

Sometimes it needs an accident in the States to make Congress press for action, though it is not certain whether that was true in this case.

Did Captain Fatally Delay Evacuation for King? (Riyadh, 1980)
All die when home and dry

> This example highlights the danger of not evacuating a burning aircraft as soon as possible. Not only was cockpit resource management (CRM) poor, or rather nonexistent, but the second officer was dyslexic and had been thumbing through the flight manual, repeating, "No problem, no problem."
>
> Saudia Flight 163, August 19, 1980

The Saudia L1011 TriStar had come in to Riyadh from Karachi, Pakistan. At about 10 p.m. it lifted off for Jeddah, in Saudi Arabia. On board were 287 passengers, 11 cabin crew, and 3 aircrew. For such a short domestic hop there would be relatively little fuel on board and no need to jettison it if an emergency landing became necessary.

It had a Saudi captain, a Saudi first officer with very limited experience of the L1011, and an American second officer, who reputedly had been a captain at the airline, but on being found to be dyslexic had been allowed to stay on as a flight engineer. One would have thought being dyslexic would be a greater handicap for an engineer than a pilot.

While climbing through fifteen thousand feet to their cruising height, the flight crew heard an alarm. A warning light indicated the presence of smoke in the rear cargo hold, C-3. This first indication of possible trouble occurred just seven minutes after takeoff.

The crew then spent some four minutes verifying the alert, with the second officer thumbing through the flight manual to find the procedure to follow.

Since they would have to double back this delay going in the wrong direction added eight minutes to the time it would take to get back to Riyadh. They had reached twenty-two thousand feet when the captain decided to return to do just that. Two minutes later the wisdom of his decision was confirmed by the presence of smoke to the rear of the passenger cabin.

Perhaps because the first officer had little experience of the L1011, the captain did not delegate tasks. He not only flew the aircraft himself but also performed the other tasks, such as communication with the cabin crew and the airport. He was undoubtedly overstretched but managed to touch down normally on the runway, despite having shut down the rear engine due to a jammed throttle lever—the fire had burned through the cables.

Unbelievably, once on the ground the captain did not try to stop the aircraft as quickly as possible but let it trundle down the runway for two minutes forty seconds. Even more unbelievably, the crew left the engines running for a further three minutes fifteen seconds after that, thus holding off the rescuers, who then found their unfamiliarity with the exits meant they could not gain access for a further twenty-three minutes.

The sequence of events was as follows. [Slight discrepancies in the timings are due to them being derived from different sources.]

In the Air

Lapsed time	Local time	
	22:08:00	Takeoff from Riyadh
00:00:00	22:14:54	C-3 cargo hold smoke alarm
00:05:06	22:20:00	Return initiated
00:07:06	22:22:00	Smoke at rear of cabin, passengers panicking
00:10:32	22:25:26	Number two throttle jams. Fire already in cabin
00:12:46	22:27:40	Captain tells all to stay seated. Passengers fighting in aisles
	Final approach	Captain tells crew *not* to Evacuate
00:21:30	22:36:24	Touchdown

On the Ground

Lapsed time	Local Time	
00:00:00	22:36:24	Touchdown
00:02:40	22:39:04	Continues down runway for two minutes forty seconds
00:05:55	22:42:18	Engines cut
00:28:38	23:05:00	Rescuers finally succeed in opening door 2R
00:31:30	23:08:00	Flash fire engulfs interior, no doubt due to ingress of oxygen

By the time the rescuers gained access, the 301 occupants were long dead. The influx of oxygen caused the fire to burn even more intensely, with the result the aircraft ended up with its upper half mostly burned away.

The captain had specifically instructed his colleagues on the flight deck not to evacuate. So confident was he that evacuation would be unnecessary, he did not even tell the cabin crew to get ready just in case. There was a final transmission after the aircraft had stopped that an evacuation was about to take place, but no one opened, or managed to open, a single exit—some said the doors could not be opened because the air pressure inside the cabin was higher than outside.

Whatever the judgmental mistakes and failures of coordination on the part of the aircrew, a better form of heat and acoustic insulation above the cargo hold might have prevented the fire propagating so rapidly. Indeed, Lockheed subsequently replaced it with high-strength glass laminate.

Then there is the question of how the fire started. Interviews recorded for a 1999 BBC Panorama TV program called *Die by Wire* suggest the fire might have been caused by the Kapton insulation used for the electric wiring.

Comments by Investigators and Others on Crew Coordination

Review of the CVR showed a serious breakdown:

1. The captain failed to delegate responsibility to the other crew members, deciding to fly the aircraft and try to assess and remedy the problem as well.

2. The first officer had very limited experience on the L1011 and did not assist the captain in flying the aircraft or monitoring communications or systems.

3. The second officer, who was thought to be dyslexic, spent nearly all his time searching through

the aircraft's operations manual, the whole time
repeating to himself "No problem."

The airline modified the procedures for coping with
such emergencies and stepped up its training for
evacuations. In addition, it made sure the C-3 baggage
areas were sealed off.

It seems incredible that with conditions bad enough for
passengers to be panicking and fighting in the aisles, the
captain did not bring the aircraft to the most immediate
stop possible and evacuate. The pilots were farthest from
the fire. One possibility is that with the captain doing
everything himself, he did not realize the seriousness of
the fire, especially as the fire warnings ceased because
the intense fire had destroyed the sensors!

Was this an instance where using video cameras to give
pilots an indication of the situation in the passenger
cabins could have been helpful?

Outraged Michael Busby "Saw It All"

In the course of reviewing and updating parts of this
book, we came across an account[1] of what happened that
day at Riyadh airport by Michael Busby, an expat, who
says he was watching from his villa nearby. He claims the
reason the captain of the L1011 went down the full three
thousand seven hundred foot (four thousand meter)
length of runway, leaving the emergency vehicles
standing-by halfway down far behind and moved off onto
a taxiway was that the Saudi king's 747 was about to take
off and was already taxiing.

According to Busby, whenever the king's aircraft was in motion, the protocol was that all other aircraft should stop. Any Saudi not complying would be given a severe prison sentence. Foreign aircrew would be summarily dismissed.

Though this would explain a lot, it is difficult to believe that such a fact, if true, would not have been given more prominence when Busby suggested it. However, companies such as Lockheed, hoping for major contracts in Saudi Arabia, might not want to go down that avenue.

Busby notes that the passengers were mostly poor Pakistani pilgrims, renowned for bringing stoves with liquid fuel with them. Whether or not that had any bearing on the fire or its propagation, their families would not have been in a position to pursue litigation, especially with their government certainly not wanting to risk offending the Saudi royal family.

A Salutary Lesson?

Elsewhere in this book we have mentioned how passengers having had to evacuate an aircraft via the emergency chutes when no fire eventually breaks out often seek damages. Would they really prefer that the crew allow them to stay on board when in doubt?

---

[1] http://www.scribd.com/doc/38040625/Death-of-An-Airplane-The-Appalling-Truth-About-Saudia-Airlines-Flight-163 Dated 2010

737 Stops with Fire Upwind (Manchester, UK, 1985)
Gentle breeze blows flames onto fuselage

> A simple matter of how the aircraft stops with respect to the wind, albeit so slight a wind as to be insignificant from a flying point of view, can determine whether passengers live or die.
>
> British Airtours Flight 28M, August 22, 1985

The first production Boeing 737 short- to medium-range airliner was delivered to Lufthansa in 1968, and after a start that was so slow Boeing even considered abandoning production and selling the design to the Japanese, the aircraft became the most prolific airliner in the Western world.

By August 22, 1985, British Airtours, a subsidiary of British Airways, was using one for a routine charter flight from Manchester, in England, to Corfu, Greece. Virtually full, with 131 passengers and 6 crew members, the 737 was already engaged in its takeoff run, with the first officer as the handling pilot, when there was a loud thud.

Assuming it was a tire blowout, the captain, Peter Terrington, ordered "Stop!" and at the same time pulled back the throttles and engaged reverse thrust. After having reached a maximum speed of 126 knots, the aircraft began to slow, with Terrington checking that the spoilers had deployed.

Terrington told his first officer, Brian Love, not to hammer the brakes, in order to limit the damage to the landing gear in the event of a blowout, and there was plenty of runway left anyway, as the decision to abort the takeoff had been taken well before V_1. The first officer, who had been applying maximum braking, duly eased up on them.

As the groundspeed fell to 85 knots some nine seconds after the thud, Terrington called the tower to inform them that they were abandoning the takeoff. Almost immediately there was a fire warning for the left-hand engine. The tower then informed them there was a "lot of fire," and that the fire appliances were on their way.

With their speed below 50 knots, Terrington queried the tower as to whether an evacuation seemed necessary. The controller replied, "I would do via the starboard side." This was merely twenty seconds after the thud and twenty-five seconds before the aircraft came to a final stop. Some six seconds later, and fourteen seconds before the aircraft eventually stopped, Terrington turned the aircraft to the right so it could exit the runway via the Link Delta taxiway. Then, just before the aircraft came to a complete halt, he told the cabin crew to evacuate from the starboard side.

However, pooled fuel on the ground was burning, and flames were already lapping the rear fuselage. When the rear right-hand door was opened, no one was able to escape from there because of the flames and, worse still, flames soon penetrated through there into the cabin. What had at first seemed to be a minor incident was quickly turning into a disaster.

Difficulty in opening other emergency doors and obstructions of one sort or another resulted in two crew members and fifty-three passengers dying, and fifteen passengers sustaining serious injuries.

Sixty-three passengers and one firefighter had minor or no injuries.

Had the cabin been better designed, had materials for furnishings produced less toxic smoke, and had the evacuation been conducted in a more orderly fashion and the aircraft not stopped with the fire upwind, perhaps everyone could have escaped.

Training material for US firefighters even cites the disaster in stressing the danger hydrogen cyanide (HCN) given off by burning plastics represents, saying: "The fire killed fifty-four people, of whom forty-seven had possibly lethal cyanide levels, while only eleven had possibly fatal levels of carbon monoxide.

Painstaking studies of the disaster led investigators to make thirty-one recommendations, many of which were at the time deemed too expensive or not worthwhile on a cost-benefit basis, partly because the cost of a passenger fatality was not the $2.5 million or more it is in the United States today.

The thirty-one recommendations included the need to bring aircraft to a stop in such a way that the wind helps rather than hinders, and modifications of the air-conditioning system to prevent the spread of fumes and flashover fires.

Allegedly, a passenger sitting next to an emergency exit was incapable of opening it, thus delaying exit from there for a crucial minute.

The late Professor Helen Muir, of the UK's Cranfield University, studied the incident and replicated the conditions in the cabin. When she offered the participants money for getting off quickly, she found they behaved as the passengers on the disaster flight had, climbing over seats and pushing others out of their way. The test suggested that the melee caused by those with a strong will to survive, with them jumping over seats and so on, resulted in far fewer people escaping overall. It seems more people escape if everyone follows the cabin crew's orders.

The underlying cause of the fire was improper cold fusion welding of a defective casing in the left engine. This was in part due to poor collaboration and poor exchange of information between the engine manufacturer (Pratt & Whitney) and British Airways.

737 Pilots Shut Down Wrong Engine (Kegworth, UK, 1989)

An early example of 737 pilots unaware of changes

> The disaster described below was once the one most often cited in pilot training as an example of how dangerous precipitous—not properly considered—action can be.
>
> British Midland Flight 92, January 8, 1989

Pilots around the world were incredulous. Some even wondered whether Boeing might have connected the instruments the wrong way around. If not, how could experienced pilots make such a mistake, confusing right with left?

Furthermore, the pilots had believed there was a fire when there wasn't one.

The early-evening British Midlands Airways flight in the new version Boeing 737 from London to Northern Ireland was at 28,300 feet and climbing under rated power toward its cruising height of 35,000 feet. Then, thirteen minutes after takeoff, there was a loud bang, followed by a thumping noise and vibration. Passengers in the rear of the aircraft were disturbed to see flashes issuing from the tailpipe of the number one engine on the left—very apparent in the wintry darkness. Smoke or something like it then started coming in through the air-conditioning.

Pilots can observe events in front of them but not nearly so easily see what is happening to the aircraft and engines behind them and must rely on their instruments in the first instance, and perhaps later on reports from cabin crew and passengers. The pilots felt the shudder and vibration and heard the noise. The captain later said he smelled and saw smoke coming in through the air-conditioning; the first officer just noticed the smell of burning.

The captain immediately disengaged the autopilot and took over control, according to standard procedure. He then asked the first officer which engine was giving trouble.

The first officer replied:

It's the lef—. It's the right one.

To which the captain replied:

Okay, throttle it back.

The captain later said he thought the smoke was coming in from the passenger cabin, and, based on his knowledge of the way the air-conditioning on the previous model of the 737 was designed, concluded the smoke must be coming from the right-hand engine.

Whatever the facts, this meant the first officer was confirming what the captain already thought. The captain gave his order to throttle back the right engine nineteen seconds after the onset of the vibrations, so we are talking about a short time frame and little opportunity for reflection or study of the instruments.

When questioned later, the first officer could not say which instrument indication made him conclude it was the right engine. From the exact words of the first officer, it would appear he was not sure but felt obliged to give an answer.

Could he have subconsciously sensed the answer the captain expected? Otherwise, why would he switch from "lef—" to "right"?

With the autothrottle disengaged, the first officer duly throttled back the right engine. One or two seconds later the vibrations seemed to decrease, seemingly confirming that the right engine had been the one producing the vibrations, when in fact the vibrations coming from the left engine decreased because it was no longer operating at full rated power, as the autothrottle was disengaged when the captain took over control manually.

The captain's and first officer's preoccupation with communications with ATC and contacting the company retarded the envisaged complete shutdown of the right engine, as the pilots were required to complete the checklist procedure together. The shutdown procedure was not initiated until two minutes seven seconds after the initial major vibration. During that time the vibration indicator showed no abnormal vibration for the right engine, which was not true for the left engine, where the vibration remained high, but not as high as initially. Indeed, just before the shutdown, the first officer remarked, "Seems we have stabilized. We've still got the smoke."

By adding the remark about the smoke, was he trying to hedge his bets with the captain? Whatever the case, it must have lessened the impact of the statement that they seemed to have stabilized. To be fair, after the shutdown of the right engine, the captain did try to review with the first officer what they had done and what symptoms they had seen, saying, "Now what indications did we actually get? . . . just rapid vibrations in the aeroplane, smoke . . ."

Unfortunately, communications from ATC cut short this review. (One of the conclusions of the subsequent inquiry was that ATC should not overload pilots in emergencies.)

They were diverting to the airline's home base, East Midlands Airport, which happened to be nearby. Unfortunately, the airport's proximity meant they had no time to reassess the situation or even monitor the functioning of the left-hand engine over an extended period of level flight. The fact that ATC told them to change frequencies only served to increase their already high workload.

They increased power on their one and only engine— according to the flight data recorder their instruments showed considerable vibration (which the pilots failed to notice)—as they leveled out for a moment and made a turn to line up with the runway and descended through three thousand feet thirteen miles from the runway.

Descending with gradually increasing flap, they put the landing gear down and set the flaps to 15 degrees. Then at nine hundred feet, with only 2.4 miles to go to touchdown (on the runway), the thrust provided by their remaining engine suddenly fell away.

The captain called for the first officer to restart the number two engine, but they were going much too slowly for a windmill start, and the failing number one engine could not provide the pressure required to restart the good engine.

The flight manual did have details of how to relight using the auxiliary power unit (APU), but this explanation only applied to the number one engine.

Given time and a very good knowledge of the system, a pilot might be able to work out a way to restart the number two using the APU. This would involve switching off the air-conditioning and other procedures, and even if the first officer had been able to accomplish this, he could not have brought the engine up to speed in time to save the aircraft. Thus, the fact that the manual lacked such an explanation did not make any difference to the outcome.

Some seventeen seconds after the loss of power from the number one engine, its fire warning system activated. However, at that juncture, lack of airspeed and height, not fire, were the captain's principal concerns. Switching on the PA, he warned the passengers and cabin crew of the imminent contact with the ground by repeating the words: "Prepare for crash landing!"

The captain hardly needed the aural ground proximity warning system (GPWS) to tell him they were below the glide slope as he raised the nose in a vain attempt at least to get over the M1 motorway (freeway), which unfortunately lay transversely in a cutting along the airport perimeter. With the stick shaker indicating they were about to stall, and their airspeed down to only 115 knots, the aircraft grazed the top of the hill lying just before the motorway cutting.

With all lift virtually gone, it lopped off the tops of the trees on the nearside face of the cutting and plunged onward and downward, so that the nose struck the foot of the incline on the far side face.

Taking into account the downward component of the trajectory, the encounter with the roughly thirty-degree-upward slope of the opposite face was equivalent to encountering an obstacle sloping at some fifty degrees head-on—at a ground speed of eighty to one hundred knots.

Though the aircraft did slither some way up the far side of the cutting, the deceleration, both vertically and horizontally, was many times more than for a crash-landing on level terrain. Indeed, the stresses imposed were so great that the rear section broke off and ended up lying upside down on top of the fuselage. Partly because the central fuel tank was empty due to it being such a short journey, and partly thanks to the rapid arrival of the airport fire services, there was no major fire.

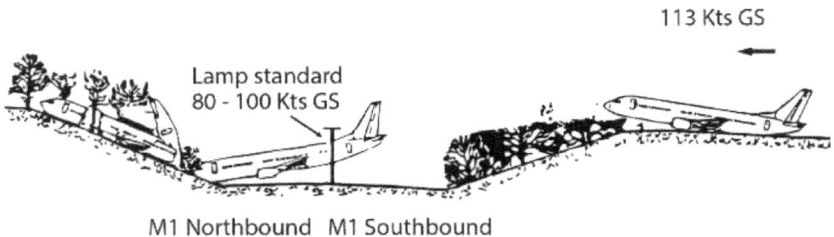

113 Kts GS

Lamp standard
80 - 100 Kts GS

M1 Northbound M1 Southbound

Kegworth impact sequence (Courtesy UK AAIB)

In total, forty-seven passengers perished, sixty-seven passengers and seven crew members were seriously injured, and four passengers and one crew member had slight or no injuries.

Though considered the classic case of what not to do, there were a number of contributory factors to what came to be called the Kegworth Air Disaster, in view of its proximity to the village of that name. These include the following:

1. False positive
   Safety expert Professor Peter Ladkin says this is the only case he is aware of where a "false positive" features in an air accident. That is to say the mistaken corrective action (shutting down the good engine) seemed to be solving the problem, thus making the pilots think they had done the right thing. This is unlike in medicine, where the long period of time over which recovery or improvement of the patient for any unrelated reason can be attributed to action by the doctor or surgeon means such false positives are well known.

   The cessation of the vibrations was one thing, but to confirm things by saying that the smoke disappeared when the pilots shut down the number two engine was, with hindsight, rather dubious thinking, since smoke would not normally disappear immediately.

2. Engine instrument system (EIS) difficult to read
   Before the introduction of two-man flight crews, the primary instruments, showing the performance of the engines were in front of the pilots, and the secondary instruments, indicating the condition of

the engines, such as oil temperature and pressure and vibration, were in front of the flight engineer. However, with the sidelining of the flight engineer, these secondary instruments had to be in front of the pilots.

In the earlier version of the aircraft, the B737-300, this was done by having traditional cockpit dials with mechanical hands, as in traditional clocks, there being two panels side by side, one with the main flying instruments, and the other showing the condition of the engines. These earlier ones with needles were easy to read at a glance.

However, as anything mechanical is liable to go wrong and anyway requires costly maintenance, LEDs were used instead of mechanical hands. However, rather than redesigning the panels to take full advantage of the virtues of an electronic display, the designers wanted to maintain the same general layout so pilots could switch from one model of the aircraft to another without expensive recertification.

In reality, LEDs could not simulate the previous clocklike hands, because those available at that time could not be bunched up at the center of the dials to look like a continuous line. Instead, the designers placed three rather pathetic-looking LEDs at intervals around the perimeter of the dials.

These could still be read by pilots with good eyesight when looking for a particular reading but made comparison and noticing anything unusual more difficult. In addition, Boeing had reduced the size of the secondary engine display relative to that for the primary display instruments.

The captain and first officer had very little experience (twenty-three and fifty-three hours respectively) on the 737-400 version, and the airline did not yet have a simulator where they could have practiced using the new engine information system (EIS), with its diodes. In addition, the captain said his considerable experience with other aircraft had led him to distrust vibration readings in general, and he did not include them in his usual scan of the instruments. His conversion training had not included instruction that technical improvements meant that spurious vibration readings were very unlikely.

3. Training and checklists

In the training of the BMA 737 pilots, the need to think or check things out before taking precipitous action was stressed, but as already mentioned there had not been training on a flight simulator with the new hybrid EIS display. There was a checklist for what to do in case of vibration from the engines and one for what to do when smoke occurred, but not one for when they happened simultaneously.

At the time pilots at BMA had not been made fully aware that there was no need to shut down engines completely because of vibration, nor that engine fans which are vibrating or not properly aligned could have their fan tips touching the rubber seals on the periphery and that this could produce smoke and a smell of burning but did not mean the engine was on fire. Thus, as the investigators said, the situation was outside the pilots' experience and training.

4. Workload and stress: Fear of fire
    In many emergencies, airlines usually insist that captains take control. Captains also tend to take control in difficult situations when it is not quite an emergency. Doing something physical makes the captain feel he is coping and relieves stress. The trouble with this is that the captain is concentrating on the physical task of flying the aircraft, or, as in the case of SQ006 at Taipei, maneuvering it over the slippery taxiway in bad visibility and heavy rain, and misses the larger picture.

    The flight data recorder (FDR) revealed that when the captain disengaged the autopilot, the aircraft yawed sixteen degrees to the left, a sign that the left engine was producing less power than the one on the right, but he did not seem to notice, as he did nothing to correct it. The fact that the first officer reported to ATC early on that they had an "emergency situation like an engine fire" shows they were concerned about fire, even though up to then none of the engine fire alarms had triggered.

    It is an interesting psychological point that a smell can instantly transport one mentally to a certain place, and the shaking of the aircraft followed by the smell of burning may have caused the pilots to react more instinctively and precipitously than they would have done in the event of a fire-warning light coming on. Anyway, a fire warning would have immediately indicated which engine had the problem.

The official report made the additional point that having another pilot take over the handling of the aircraft—as PF (pilot flying)—meant monitoring of the instruments was less consistent than it might have been.

Up until the onset of the vibration, the first officer had been flying the aircraft and would have been concentrating on the main instruments, not the engine vibration indicator, it being the role of the PNF (pilot not flying; in this case the captain, who did not believe in scanning vibration readings) to do the general monitoring. The captain must have thought the first officer had good reason to say it was the right engine that was giving trouble.

5. Unfortunate timing.

    The pilots did not have the height or speed to restart the good engine, and not enough height to choose a flat place to land. Had the airport been farther away, they would have had found the problems with the number one engine when still high enough to restart the other one.

6. Passengers and three cabin crew knew

    Passengers at the rear who had seen the "sparks"

from the left engine when the initial trouble occurred were somewhat perplexed when the captain said he had shut down the right engine but did not inform the cabin crew because the captain sounded supremely confident.

The three members of the cabin crew who had also seen the sparks apparently did not notice the captain saying the right engine had been shut down. They knew the purpose of the announcement was to reassure the passengers and were no doubt extremely busy with their own duties as they got ready for the unexpected landing.

A retired British Airways flight attendant has suggested to the author that the failure to pick up on the captain's mistake might have come about because cabin staff themselves often get confused about left and right, as they face backwards when addressing the passengers.

Just after shutdown of the number two engine, the captain called the flight service manager (FSM) to the flight deck to tell him to clear things for landing, and at the same time asked him, "Did you get smoke in the cabin back there?" He got the reply "We did. Yes."

This perhaps only confirmed the captain's mistaken view that the right-hand engine must have been at fault. The FSM departed but returned a minute later to say the passengers were panicky, and it was only then that the captain announced to the passengers that a little trouble with the right engine had produced some smoke, but it would be okay, as they had shut it down, and would be landing about ten minutes thereafter.

Cause of the Engine Problem

Subsequent studies showed a vibration harmonic at certain speeds of rotation caused the fan blades to rub against the rubber seals on the periphery, producing the burning smell and causing one blade to break. The manufacturer rectified the harmonic problem and allowed extra space between the blades and the seals to give a greater safety margin, should such vibration reoccur.

Other Similar Incidents

Before these modifications, other 737s with the same engine, including a BMA 737, had similar engine problems when climbing at maximum rated power. Benefiting from the lessons learned from the previous incident, the crews immediately studied the vibration indicator and made sure they shut down the correct engine before landing safely. They then used a lower power rating, until the manufacturer modified the engines as described above.

This was not an in-flight fire at all. Though the first officer had cited the possibility of an engine fire, the instruments did not give a fire warning until the number one engine failed just prior to the crash. As so often when pilots have been partially responsible for a crash, the airline first defended them and then let them go.

Rearward-Facing Seats?

The high number of fatalities and injuries in what was a crash at relatively low speed led the authorities to examine the safety aspects of the seating, the strength of the flooring, and the locking of the overhead lockers. Some asked whether rear-facing seating might have offered greater protection.

The comprehensive official report said rear-facing seating could impose too great a stress on cabin flooring, adding that rearward-facing seats:

1. Could be less effective in accidents in which the main deceleration force is not along the longitudinal axis of the aircraft.

2. Could expose occupants to the risk of injury from loose objects in an accident.

3. And great improvements had been made in the design and construction of forward-facing seats.

4. May not be suitable for use in modern jets, with their high climb-out angles, and they could be "psychologically less attractive to passengers."

Fierce Oxygen-fed Fire in ValuJet Cargo Hold (Everglades, 1996)
Fire so strong it melted the cabin floor

> This disaster received much publicity not only because of its gravity but also because passengers shouting "Fire... Fire!" could be heard on the CVR recording.
>
> ValueJet Flight 592, May 11, 1996

The subtropical Everglades National Park, in Southern Florida, is said to be the only place in the world where alligators and crocodiles cohabit. Much of it consists of swamp interspersed with strips of shallow water filled with vegetation, with mud at the bottom.

A worse place for recovering the bodies and debris from an air crash would be difficult to find. Not only were the hot and humid working conditions particularly difficult for people in protective suits, but it was also hard to locate the evidence and body parts in the ooze. The only good news for the investigators was that the shock wave, while attracting alligators, had scared away poisonous snakes.

ValuJet Flight 592, a DC-9 with 105 passengers, 3 cabin crew, and 2 pilots, had just taken off in the early afternoon from Miami International Airport for Atlanta and climbed through ten thousand feet when the pilots heard a strange sound. No sooner had they concluded it was from an electrical bus than other electrical problems manifested themselves.

Shortly afterward, shouts of "Fire... Fire," presumably from the passenger cabin, could be heard on the CVR.

The thirty-five-year-old female captain of the DC-9, Candalyn Kubeck, did not declare a Mayday but radioed the Miami International Airport controller, saying an immediate return to Miami was required.

The controller, not grasping the situation, twice gushed on with the instructions for the routine handover to Miami Center. Once her words had sunk in, he lost no time giving her a heading and a height (seven thousand feet) to return to Miami and asked for the nature of the problem. Kubeck told him it was smoke in the cabin and in the cockpit.

Shortly afterward she asked if there was an airport even nearer but continued to be vectored to Miami, perhaps because there was not deemed to be one suitable. Anyway, it became academic, as radio communication with the aircraft was then lost.

Captain Kubeck had more than two thousand hours' experience on the aircraft type, and nine thousand flying hours in total. Neither her ability nor that of her first officer, Richard Hazen, a fifty-two-year-old ex–air force pilot, could have made any difference to the subsequent outcome, an event sometimes referred to as the "ValuJet situation," where an extremely fierce fire in a vulnerable part of the aircraft is only detected a few seconds before the aircraft becomes uncontrollable.

In this case, *only forty-nine seconds* had elapsed from the first hint of trouble to the moment someone opened the flight deck door and said, "Okay, we need oxygen; we can't get oxygen back there."

The following extract from the CVR, with some standard acknowledgements omitted for brevity, gives a good idea of how the situation evolved.

Elapsed time	Local time	
–6:54	14:04:09	Takeoff from Miami (V_R)
0:00	14:10:03	Strange noise heard in cockpit: probably that of tire bursting in the hold.
0:04	14:10:07	Captain: What's that?
0:05	14:10:08	FO: I don't know.
0:09	14:10:12	Captain: [??] 'bout to lose a bus.[1]
0:12	14:10:15	FO: We got some electrical problem.
0:14	14:10:17	FO: Yeah. That battery charger's kicking in. We gotta...
0:17	14:10:20	Captain: We're losing everything.
0:18	14:10:21	Departure control gives frequency for handover to Miami Center.
0:19	14:10:22	Captain: We need to go back to Miami.
0:20	14:10:23	Shouts from passenger cabin.
0:22	14:10:25	Female voices shout: Fire ... Fire ... Fire
0:24	14:10:27	We're on fire! (repeated)
0:26	14:10:29	Departure control repeats Instructions for handover to Miami Center.
0:29	14:10:32	R/T first officer to departure: 592 needs immediate return to Miami.
0:32	14:10:35	Departure control: Roger, turn left heading 270, descend and maintain seven thousand.
0:38	14:10:41	Departure control asks what kind of problem they are having and is informed it is smoke in the cockpit and cabin.
0:49	14:10:52	Sound of cockpit door moving.
0:55	14:10:58	Third cockpit microphone: Okay, we need oxygen. We can't get oxygen back there.

1:04	14:11:07	Departure control: When able, turn left heading 250, descend and maintain five thousand. (592 acknowledges.)
1:09	14:11:12	Third cockpit microphone: Completely on fire.
1:11	14:11:14	Shouting from passenger cabin subsides, perhaps because occupants are overcome by smoke.
1:18	14:11:21	Loud sound like rushing air—cockpit window opened?
1:35	14:11:38	R/T FO to departure control: 592, we need the closest airport available.
1:39	14:11:42	Departure control does not propose another airport; says they (Miami) will be standing by and 592 can plan for Runway 12.
	14:11:45	One-minute-fifteen-second interruption to CVR.
	14:12:48	[CVR stops recording.]
2:54	14:12:57	[CVR restarts.] Loud sound of rushing air?
2:55	14:12:58	Departure controller tells 592 to contact Miami approach, correctly telling them to remain on his frequency.
3:08	14:13:11	CVR recording interrupted for unknown period.
		CVR restarts for a moment. Apart from a radio transmission from an unknown source, one can only briefly hear the loud sound of rushing air. Recording ends.
	14:13:34	Total loss of control is evident from the trajectory of the aircraft. (Pilot incapacitation/aircraft uncontrollable.)
	14:13:42	Impact with ground (radar data).

Situation in the Aircraft and Impact

For the passenger cabin to be completely on fire (and not just filling with smoke) after one minute, nine seconds' elapsed time shows just how quickly the situation got out of hand.

In fact, after melting the electrical cables, the fire was eating away at the steel control cables needed to maneuver the aircraft. The aircraft then keeled over, plunged downward, seemed to try to right itself for a moment, perhaps due to action by the pilots or autopilot, and then continued nose-downward into the swamp below.

The force of the impact was such that both the aircraft and passengers ended up as a dispersed collection of difficult-to-recover pieces. All 110 people on board would have died instantly on impact if they had not already succumbed due to the fire and noxious smoke.

The Investigation

By a stroke of luck—a searcher stepped on it—the flight data recorder (FDR) was soon found and, with the cockpit voice recorder (CVR), was retrieved from the swamp.

Together with the evidence from the Miami ATC recordings, they confirmed that fire had brought about the crash. In addition, the debris showed the fire had been limited to the forward cargo hold and the area immediately above, thus making the usual painstaking piecing together of the entire mud-encrusted aircraft irrelevant.

For a fire in a hold to set the cabin above on fire, it had to have penetrated the cabin floor. In fact, some of the aluminum used in the construction of the passengers' seats was found to have melted, showing the temperature even there must have reached 1,200°F (650°C) before the aircraft cooled down on hitting the watery swamp.

Investigators later established that the temperature in that hold could have reached 3,000°F (1,600°C).

Not only had these high temperatures deformed and melted the floor separating the cargo hold from the passenger cabin, but they had first fused the electrical cables (the first anomaly the pilots noticed) and then the steel cables essential for controlling the aircraft.

This would have made it impossible for the pilots to pull the aircraft out of its precipitous dive into the swamp, assuming they were still able to function.

Oddly, the hold in question was a Class D hold and virtually airtight, so that any fire ignited there would normally soon consume the available oxygen and die down, and in the absence of a fire-extinguishing system would only smolder, at least until someone opened the hatch, which would be on the ground.

This led to the following two questions:

1. What had ignited the fire?
2. Where had oxygen come from?

As study of the cargo manifest soon revealed, it must have been the five boxes of discarded oxygen generators loaded there.

There were also three tires, at least two of which were mounted on wheels and hence liable to burst violently if overheated in a fire.

These oxygen generators came from three secondhand MD-80 aircraft that were being modified and checked out at Miami by SabreTech, a large contractor responsible for ValuJet's line and heavy maintenance. ValuJet had purchased these aircraft to upgrade and improve its fleet.

Oxygen generators supply oxygen to passengers should the cabin depressurize. These consist of canisters placed *at intervals* in the fascia above passengers that produce oxygen by an exothermic (heat-producing) chemical reaction triggered by a spring-loaded firing pin striking an explosive percussion cap. A lanyard pulls out the retaining pin when emergency oxygen is required.

On firing to provide oxygen, the temperature of the canister shell can reach between 475 and 500°F (246 to 260°C), but this heat soon dissipates if the canisters are placed individually with clearance for air around them. However, having dozens of them piled together in a cardboard box and surrounded by Bubble Wrap with nowhere for the heat to go other than into neighboring canisters could produce a chain reaction should one fire accidentally.

The canisters loaded into that hold should have been fitted with safety caps to prevent such accidental firing.

Furthermore, the ramp agent present in the cargo hold as the boxes were loaded heard a clink and objects moving around inside one of the boxes, which were stowed on top of the tires without restraints to ensure they stayed in place. Possibly that box could have fallen off.

Probable Cause

The National Transportation Safety Board (NTSB) determined that the probable causes of the accident, which resulted from a fire in the airplane's Class D cargo compartment, initiated by the actuation of one or more oxygen generators being improperly carried as cargo, were:

1. The failure of SabreTech to properly prepare, package, and identify unexpended chemical oxygen generators before presenting them to ValuJet for carriage.

2. The failure of ValuJet to properly oversee its contract maintenance program to ensure compliance with maintenance, maintenance training, and hazardous materials requirements and practices.

3. The failure of the Federal Aviation Administration (FAA) to require smoke detection and fire suppression systems in Class D cargo compartments.

Contributing to the accident:

1. The failure of the FAA to adequately monitor ValuJet's heavy maintenance programs and responsibilities, including ValuJet's oversight of its contractors and SabreTech's repair station certificate.

2. The failure of the FAA to respond adequately to prior chemical oxygen generator fires with programs to address the potential hazards.

3. ValuJet's failure to ensure that both ValuJet and contract maintenance facility employees were aware of the carrier's no-carry hazardous materials policy and had received appropriate hazardous materials training.

Incidentally, those horrifying words on the CVR so shocked Congress, as well as the public, that criticism of the FAA became especially harsh.

Had the FAA made the installation of fire detectors and fire-suppressant systems mandatory for such Class D cargo holds, the pilots might well have been able to bring the aircraft back to Miami before things got out of hand.

An interesting point was that the maintenance workers doing twelve-hour shifts **were** concerned about the safety aspect, but their focus was on the safety of the MD-80s they were working on!

William Langewiesche has covered this organizational accident in detail in the March 1998 edition of the *Atlantic Monthly*, referring to the work on the prevention of such accidents carried out by academics. Incidentally, he adds that some academics claim the extra safety features incorporated into systems can in themselves lead to accidents, as in the Chernobyl nuclear disaster and here in the ValuJet case.

---

[1] Fundamental electric power distributor. (See note for Swissair on-board fire.)

The TWA-800 Controversy (JFK Outbound, 1996)
How could so many witnesses be wrong?

> No other air crash has engendered so much speculation about conspiracies. We include it in this chapter because the sheer scale of the cover-up required would inevitably have resulted in leaks via whistle-blowers.
>
> TWA Flight 800, July 17, 1996

The twenty-five-year-old Boeing 747 for Trans World Airlines Flight TWA-800 to Paris had arrived at New York's JFK International Airport from Athens at 16:31 on July 17, 1996.

After cleaning and servicing, it was due to depart for the French capital at 19:00, but because of a delay, caused mainly by confusion over whether a passenger's suitcase was on board and not the passenger, it did not depart until 20:03.

The air conditioners were not needed when cleaners and mechanics started servicing the aircraft, but the extra hour's wait with passengers on board at the end and the hot conditions meant they were working hard for about two and a half hours prior to departure and pumping out a great amount of heat.

The fuel in the center-wing fuel tank would normally have absorbed some of this heat, but as that was virtually empty, since relatively little fuel was required for the short hop across the Atlantic to Paris, the temperature of that tank would have risen significantly. The tank would have been full of easily ignited fumes.

At 20:18 the aircraft was cleared for takeoff. The climb-out from JFK over the sea proceeded as usual. Then, passing under the control of the Boston Air Route Control Center, it received various instructions regarding its flight level. Up until then the only thing of note was the captain saying: "Look at that crazy fuel flow indicator there on number four . . . See that?"

One minute later Boston Center told them to climb from Flight Level 130 to Flight Level 150. As they were complying, there was a loud sound, after which the CVR stopped working (20:31:12).

With many aircraft in the general area, Boston Center received several reports from pilots about witnessing an explosion, with the most detailed being that of the captain of an Eastwind Airlines Boeing 737: "Saw an explosion out here . . . Ahead of us here . . . About 16,000 feet [4,900 meters] or something like that. It just went down into the water."

The debris had fallen into the sea in a busy area a few miles off the coast, and it was only a matter of minutes before people in all sorts of craft, both military and civilian, were on the scene. Fuel was burning on the water. As feared, there were no survivors, making the death toll 230.

There was much suspicion that the aircraft had been blown up by a terrorist bomb or shot down by a US missile, or even some secret ray gun under test.

A respected CIA agent (now deceased) told someone the author knows personally that on reviewing the TWA 800 radar tracks, he right away thought it was distinctly possible that it had been shot down by a US missile. Nothing sinister in this, he would have thought, as accidents do happen.

The Investigation

This was the most time-consuming and painstaking investigation carried out by the NTSB. There was some friction with the FBI, who took the lead initially when it was assumed to be the result of a terrorist act.

The FBI did exhaustive checks of logs and so forth to make sure no US Navy vessel could have been involved. They also interviewed the many witnesses, some of whom seemed to think they saw a missile going up and striking the aircraft. However, the FBI did not record the witnesses' actual words and only summed up what they said.

Much of the NTSB's work involved disproving that such and such—say a missile or bomb—could have been the cause. They laboriously pieced together a twenty-seven-meter (ninety-foot) section of the aircraft and were able to work out the way the aircraft had broken up.

Though traces of explosive residue were found, their locations were *never* associated with evidence of an explosion. Also, there were various explanations for their presence, including their being a "leftover" from an exercise using sniffer dogs to look for explosives, or contamination from navy ships and from the clothes of military personnel.

Conclusion

The NTSB concluded that an explosion in the center fuel tank was the cause. Despite the equipment in the tank for measuring the amount of fuel employing voltages too low to cause ignition, a short circuit in wiring outside might have led to an overvoltage in wires leading to that equipment. The recovered fuel-quantity indicator showed 640 pounds when only 300 had been loaded, a reading that could have been caused by the overvoltage. Two and a half minutes before the disaster, the captain had mentioned "crazy" readings for the number four engine fuel-flow gauge, suggesting some electrical anomaly.

The NTSB had not been happy with the idea of only relying on avoiding ignition sources in the fuel tank in the early 747-100s as the sole means of protection and thought having the air-conditioning dissipating so much excess heat into the tank was undesirable.

To lessen the risk, it was decided the empty space should in future be filled with an inert gas.

Could So Many Witnesses Be Wrong?

The rumor mill was fed by the witness reports, with some saying something went up towards the aircraft. The fact that the FBI were very cagey and only belatedly released their summaries and hid identities raised suspicions.

Air crash investigators well know how witnesses can be unreliable. More credence was given to the Eastwind Airlines Boeing 737 captain who saw TWA-800 *merely* explode.

Swissair 111 Cockpit Fire (JFK Outbound, 1998)

Was the flight entertainment system responsible?

> Investigators recommended that aircrew be made aware of the need to land as quickly as possible in the case of potentially serious onboard fires. Any delay incurred due to the desire to dump fuel is liable to close the narrow window of opportunity to save the aircraft and the lives of those on board.
>
> Swissair Flight SR111, September 2, 1998

Swissair Flight SR111 had taken off from New York's JFK Airport en route for Geneva at 18:17, with 215 passengers and 14 crew members. The aircraft was a McDonnell Douglas MD-11, a trijet that had evolved from the DC-10, with the addition of much automation to dispense with the need for a flight engineer.

A more logical name might have been the DC-11, but one can understand the manufacturer's hesitation to suggest it was a DC-10+. Actually, the famous DC designation stood simply for the rather unglamorous-sounding "Douglas Commercial" and MD fitted the company name similarly.

Following the great circle route to Western Europe, skirting Canada's eastern seaboard, the MD-11 was some sixty-six nautical miles from Halifax and at thirty-three thousand feet when the crew alerted Monckton Center (Monckton high level controller) that a serious situation was developing, but not one that could be classed as an emergency. They did this by using the words "Pan, Pan, Pan" instead of "Mayday, Mayday, Mayday."

Swissair 111 heavy is declaring Pan, Pan, Pan.

We have smoke in the cockpit. Request deviate immediate right turn to a convenient place—I guess Boston. We need first the weather so uh we start a right turn here.

As Boston was then three hundred nautical miles away, and Halifax International Airport only sixty-six nautical miles away, the Monckton controller asked whether they would prefer to go to Halifax, to which SR111 agreed, and began descending from thirty-three thousand feet. The controller informed them that the active runway at Halifax was 06 and went on to ask whether they wanted a vector for it. SR111 answered in the affirmative and was told to turn left onto the north-northeast course of thirty degrees.

There were a number of exchanges with controllers and even a British Airways aircraft listening-in regarding the weather at Halifax. This indicated the pilots thought they had adequate time, and the situation was not critical.

When the Halifax controller subsequently informed them they had thirty miles to go to the runway threshold, SR111 surprisingly demurred, saying:

We need more than thirty miles . . .

The controller instructed them to turn left and to lose some altitude, and SR111 confirmed they were turning left.

SR111 called the controller:

We must dump some fuel. We may do that in this area during descent.

The controller said "Okay," whereupon SR111 told him they could turn left or right toward the south to dump fuel. The controller told them to make what was in effect a U-turn to the left and to inform him when they were ready to dump. They duly made the U-turn.

There were various exchanges regarding the fuel dump and the range of altitude over which it could be done.

Before they could begin the dump, the situation suddenly became desperate.

Swissair SR111:

> *Swissair one eleven heavy is declaring emergency. We are between uh twelve and five thousand feet we are declaring emergency now at ah time ah zero one two four.*

Confirming their clearance to commence dumping fuel on that track, the controller asked to be informed when the fuel dump was completed. He called again, repeating his authorization to dump.

Some six minutes after that, the aircraft struck the water after having made a 360-degree turn. All 229 persons on board lost their lives.

How did the situation deteriorate so quickly? Or was it more serious than thought right from the beginning?

The Final Report

The 352-page final report of the Canadian Transport Safety Bureau can be found via their website, ***http://tsb.gc.ca/***. It has much general technical information about wiring, highly automated aircraft systems, and measures to prevent and deal with onboard fires. Anyone especially interested in this accident should consult the report directly.

To sum it up rather inadequately:

1. Aircraft manufacturers, regulators, operators, and pilots do not normally consider smoke or fumes issuing from the air-conditioning system to represent a serious and immediate emergency requiring an immediate landing. For example, in the British Midland accident in which the pilots shut down the wrong engine, the "smoke" exiting the air-conditioning came from the engine fan blades rubbing the rubber seals and did not represent a fire at all.

2. The Swissair crew initially thought it was something affecting the air-conditioning and went through the checklist for that and, reasonably, did not think it was a dire emergency; hence, the use of "Pan, Pan, Pan" rather than "Mayday."

3. The fire started in an inaccessible place in the cockpit, where there was wiring, and involved wiring for the entertainment system. Instead of being connected to a bus dedicated to passenger facilities, the entertainment system, which used a considerable amount of power, was connected to a main bus. When the pilots eventually realized the problem must be electrical in nature, various instruments and equipment were already failing, and they had to fly manually.

4. Contrary to early reports, the pilots could not have reached Halifax even had they opted to come

straight in from the moment they declared "Pan, Pan, Pan."

5. Though there was a sign of arcing (spark between wires) on the cable for the in-flight entertainment system cable in the area where the fire started, there was no proof that it was this that actually started the fire.

NTSB Recommendations

"We recommend that the Safety Regulation Group reiterates its advice to airlines that the priority in certain emergencies, such as in-flight fires, is to land rather than to seek to dump fuel in order to avoid an overweight landing.

It should ensure through its inspections that airlines are passing on that information to aircrews.

Furthermore, we recommend that air traffic controllers be given similar advice so that they are able to respond appropriately to such emergencies."

Cockpit Fires

While any onboard fire is potentially a great hazard, those in the cockpit can be particularly pernicious as they can incapacitate the pilots as well as compromise the controls.

One theory is that it may have been a factor in the mysterious disappearance in 2014 of Malaysia Airlines Flight MH370 that took off from Kuala Lumpur for Beijing only to deviate from its course shortly after departure and end up somewhere in the sea off Australia with no communication from the pilots.

In 2016, the crash of an EgyptAir A320 may also have been due to a cockpit fire with some suggestions it was started by the copilot's mobile phone or tablet, though others think the fire more likely started in the avionics bay just below.

Fragmenting Tire Dooms Supersonic Concorde (Paris-CDG, 2000)

Almost certainly overweight

> The Anglo-French supersonic Concorde, the most glamorous and most beautiful airliner ever, stirred the hearts of the public in France and the UK, who had paid out so much in taxes to support it and its wealthy passengers.
>
> Air France Flight 4590, July 25, 2000

Concorde's History

The world's first supersonic airliner, the Concorde 001, rolled onto the tarmac in 1967, but according to CNN it took two more years of testing and fine-tuning of the powerful engines before it made its maiden flight over France on March 2, 1969.

The original plan was for a production run of three hundred, but in the end, it was limited to just fourteen. Air France cannibalized one of those for spare parts in 1982, and another crashed, leaving five for Air France and seven for British Airways when the two airlines withdrew Concorde from service in 2003.

These days the authorities would never certify such a noisy bird, so Concorde was surviving on the certificates issued in the 1970s. Even then the United States would not approve inland flights, so its regular scheduled flights to the States were mostly to the East Coast, and New York in particular. Some said it was sour grapes at being beaten to the post on the part of the United States.

When Concorde finally entered airline service, it was a Pyrrhic victory for its makers or, rather, the two nations of taxpayers who provided such generous funding. Key countries on major overland routes refused to allow it to pass over their territories. For timesaving reasons, it was essential to fly overland, as the aircraft did not have the range to fly the long routes over the Pacific Ocean. Finally, the fuel-guzzling Concorde had the misfortune to come on the scene just as fuel prices were skyrocketing.

The majestic Concorde mainly benefited the rich and famous, though many found first class on a conventional aircraft to be preferable to the cramped seating on Concorde. Some celebrities, such as the British TV personality David Frost, were virtually commuting between London and New York on Concorde.

Not so well known is the good use courier companies, such as DHL, put it to in delivering documents and financial instruments for major companies when time really was money. Even so, not enough demand existed to employ fully even that tiny fleet.

Air France had more difficulty filling seats than British Airways, who made a healthy profit out of it. Not only was this because more top business people and celebrities fly to London but also partly because London is nearer than Paris to New York and Washington—quite significant with an aircraft operating near the limit of its operating range. Air France used charter flights and excursions to help fill those seats.

The Fatal Flight

Indeed, the flight that was to last only a minute or two before ending in disaster just after taking off from Paris's Charles de Gaulle Airport in July 2000 was just such a charter flight. It carried elderly Germans to New York to join a luxury Caribbean cruise.

Concorde spooled up its engines to take off with its long beak tipped five degrees downward and pointing just in front of another Air France aircraft, which had brought the French president and his wife back from an official visit to Japan. (The nose usually droops down five degrees for takeoff, and twelve-and-a-half degrees on landing, so the long nose does not obscure the pilots' view.) Though slim and elegant, the Concorde was almost certainly overweight, with fuel representing just over half her total weight.

The captain *thought* they had an all-up weight (AUW) of 185,100 kilos, placing them, he said, at the aircraft's structural limit. He did not know this was an underestimate[1] and did not include nineteen items of baggage loaded at the last minute. It is also likely that the unburned fuel in the rear tank and the nineteen extra items of luggage had moved the center of gravity too far aft.

Much to the surprise of the BEA (Bureau d'Enquêtes et d'Analyses, the French Air Accident Investigation Bureau), the announcement by the control tower of an eight-knot tailwind did not elicit any comment from the aircrew.

At the very least, the captain should have considered taking off against the wind. Although a wind of eight knots may not seem much, taking off in the opposite direction would mean sixteen knots less groundspeed. Because of limitations on the maximum speed for the tires, a tail wind of eight knots meant they were too heavy.

An article in the British Sunday newspaper the *Observer*, written by David Rose shortly after the crash, with comments by veteran Concorde pilot John Hutchinson, said they could no doubt have "got away" with being overweight had other things not gone wrong. The crew had decided 150 knots should be V_1, the speed at which they would be committed to continuing the takeoff, and 183 knots should be V_R, the speed at which they would rotate and expect to soar into the sky.

A supersonic delta-wing aircraft like Concorde differs from other aircraft in that the wings do not provide any real lift before rotation. In consequence, the tires continue to bear the entire weight of the aircraft throughout the takeoff run. This in turn means they are particularly vulnerable just before rotation, as there is not only the weight of the aircraft to consider but also the tremendous centrifugal forces acting on their treads due to the wheels' high rate of rotation. In addition, at such high speeds sharp objects on the runway are far more likely to cut into them.

Shortly after Concorde had reached V_1, the right-hand tire on the left-hand main landing gear ran over a curved strip of metal that had just fallen off a DC-10 that had taken off shortly before. Curved like a loop, the titanium strip was lying sideways up, with its concave side facing the oncoming tire, thus ensuring the tire would trap it rather than roll it over and bend it flat. The tough metal sliced into the tire, causing the tire to break up under the enormous centrifugal forces. Later, investigators found a 10 lb (4.5 kg) piece of rubber from the tire on the runway near that point.

After complex studies the BEA investigators concluded the lump of rubber had forcefully struck the underside of the wing, pushing it and the fuel tank so rapidly inward that it induced a shock wave in the fuel of such intensity that, with the tank virtually full and no air-filled spaces to absorb the shock, the tank ruptured elsewhere, a phenomenon that had never been seen before in a passenger aircraft. Had the piece of rubber just pierced the tank, as in a previous instance in Washington in 1979, the damage to the tank would doubtless have been less.

From the amount of fuel on the runway and other evidence, it is estimated that kerosene was pouring out from under the wing at a rate of sixty kilos a second. In the Washington incident above, the fuel did not catch fire, and the aircraft was able to take off and return safely. Perhaps because of the much greater amount of fuel, and very likely because a damaged wire in the landing gear was producing sparks, the leaking fuel then caught fire.

The events leading to the ultimate disaster all happened in some three seconds and must have been very confusing to the crew. The control tower told the Concorde's crew they had flames coming out behind them. Debris, and more likely hot gases from the fire, caused the performance of the two engines on the left side to fall off, resulting in a yaw to the left. The captain rotated the aircraft early as they deviated to the left of the runway, but no sooner had they lifted off than the fire warning for the number two engine sounded and the flight engineer shut it down.

The number one engine seemed to be recovering and able to help them reach the 220-knot speed to fly at least horizontally with the landing gear down. They tried to raise the landing gear but were unsuccessful, no doubt due to damage caused by the fire or debris. They attained a height of two hundred feet, still with insufficient airspeed.

The number one engine began to fail, and with the first officer constantly warning them about the lack of airspeed, the aircraft went slightly nose-up, and the left wing dropped down to 115 degrees. The yaw and sideslip meant air was no longer properly entering the good engines on the right-hand side, and they too lost power, though it is possible they were throttled back at the last minute in an attempt to straighten the aircraft's trajectory.

Virtually upside down, the pride of France and Britain crashed on a two-star hotel some six kilometers from the end of the runway and exploded in a fireball.

The crash was so violent with debris scattered widely, that there was no hope of survivors.

The death toll was a hundred passengers, six cabin attendants, and three aircrew.

Fortunately, the three-story hotel was almost empty, and on the ground "only" four people were killed and six injured. Forty-five Polish tourists staying at the hotel later returned from sightseeing to find a surprising sight.

Conclusions

Although it does not say so in so many words, the lengthy BEA report into the crash gives the impression the Air France Concorde team of officials, mechanics, and aircrew were an exclusive lot, like those associated with expensive racing cars, and had a somewhat cavalier attitude. With such cars, drivers are liable to take risks when overtaking in the belief that the tremendous reserve of power will always get them out of difficulties, and with the Concorde allow taking off in a tailwind.

As already mentioned, the extra distance to New York from Paris meant that Concorde would often be operating just within its safety envelope as regards fuel. To give that little bit extra and lessen the likelihood of being unable to reach New York, the Concorde would often be loaded with excess fuel on the assumption (or pretext) that taxiing would use it up before takeoff.

Just after the accident, maintenance staff who had replaced part of the thrust reverser mechanism on one of the engines became so distressed at the thought they might have been responsible for the disaster that they had to go to the doctor for medication. One can imagine the anguish they endured until it was discovered that the accident was unconnected with their work, carried out properly.

However, as mentioned the BEA investigators did find other maintenance workers had forgotten a spacer when reassembling the landing gear during earlier servicing.

An article appeared in the British *Observer* newspaper suggesting that omission of the spacer had caused the aircraft to deviate to the left and that the lack of it only made matters worse when the tire failed, causing the aircraft to veer to the left "like a supermarket trolley with a jammed wheel." The BEA disputed this, saying the aircraft only started to deviate when the thrust from two engines on the left-hand side fell away.

While saying the lack of the spacer had not played any role in the accident scenario, the BEA was unhappy about this evidence of maintenance failures and lack of written material showing procedures had been signed off on completion. It noted that the Air France maintenance people justified working twelve-hour shifts by claiming this avoided wasting time briefing others.

The BEA inquiry took extra time because it was run in parallel with, but separately from, the judicial inquiry, which in the end did not come up with anything dramatic. Some of the investigators from England complained it took a long time to see the evidence, and the BEA report has a note saying that this was due to the judicial inquiry.

The Insurers

The French insurers were very pleased to have come to an amicable albeit expensive agreement with the relatives of the German victims, as they wanted to avoid litigation in US courts.

However, the lawyers for the other victims' relatives were not as happy with this quick settlement and asked for extra compensation for their own services.

Could the Aircraft have been Saved?

While the direct cause of the accident was running over the titanium strip, there were suggestions that the crew might well have been able to save the aircraft had it not been overloaded, with the center of gravity too far aft, and had the flight engineer not shut down the number two engine.

However, the intensity of the fire was so great that the left wing and associated control systems would have failed before reaching the nearby Le Bourget Airport. Indeed, there is evidence that failure of the left elevon was what caused the left wing to drop at the end. Aluminum loses much of its strength when heated to a mere three hundred degrees Celsius and melts at six hundred degrees, and investigators found molten aluminum under the flight path.

One point that the BEA investigators did make about safety in general was that when something is used so little, improvements do not tend to be made. This applied to the tires, for if there had been hundreds of Concordes in operation, developing much safer tires would surely have been thought worthwhile.

When Concorde returned to service, it had new NZG^2 tires, developed by Michelin, which had new materials making them more resistant to foreign bodies and designed so that only small pieces would fly off if they did happen to fail.

In addition, the fuel tanks were lined with Kevlar, used for body armor, impregnated with Viton, an expensive synthetic rubber able to withstand high temperatures. Thus, even in the unlikely event of a large piece of rubber flying off the newly developed tires, hitting the underside of the wing, the shock wave produced in a virtually full tank would not create a gaping hole elsewhere.

Previous Incidents

There had been a close shave, not widely publicized at the time (late 1970s), when the engine on a British Airways Concorde caught fire. The passengers escaped via the emergency slides without too much difficulty, except that a passenger wearing shoes with high heels slit the fabric of one of the slides on her way down. A male, and presumably heavier, passenger following her went right through the aperture and found himself with a sore spine on the ground below.

More troubling was the discovery later that the titanium shield above the engine, destined to protect the fuel tanks, had begun to bubble due to the intense heat of the fire. Had more time elapsed, even titanium would have failed, and there would have been an enormous conflagration. Strangely, there is no mention of this in the individual histories of any of the British Airways aircraft.

The criminal investigation run in parallel with the BEA investigation also concluded that the training of Air France's Concorde aircrew had "weaknesses," which led among other things to the shutdown of an engine before necessary. However, these various failings did not amount to gross negligence or criminal responsibility.

On July 4, 2008, a French judge agreed with a prosecutor's submission that John Taylor, the Continental mechanic who allegedly fitted the nonstandard strip, Stanley Ford, a Continental maintenance official, and the airline itself stand trial for involuntarily causing death and injuries. Also cited for trial were Henri Perrier, seventy-seven, the director of the first Concorde program, and Claude Frantzen, sixty-nine, a former director of technical services at the DGAC, the French civil aviation authority. They were alleged to have known that the Concorde's wing with its fuel tanks was fragile and vulnerable to damage from the outside.

In the end the indictments led nowhere.

---

[1] After the accident, the BEA estimated her actual takeoff weight including the 19 extra items of luggage to have been 186,451 kg. This was likely to have been an underestimate, as 20.7 kg was the average for the 103 items on the load sheet, and 84 kg was taken to be the average passenger weight including carry-on luggage. Both averages seem low for this atypical passenger profile.

[2] NZG stands for Near Zero Growth, meaning they hardly grow at all at very high rotational speeds. Michelin's work was not wasted as their new tires are being considered (along with Bridgestone's) for use with the giant Airbus A380.

China Airlines 737 Catches Fire at Stand (Okinawa, 2007)
All down to a loose bolt puncturing fuel tank

> Once an aircraft comes to a halt at the stand, passengers assume all they risk thereafter is falling down the stairs as they disembark.
>
> However, brakes and engine components may well be still hot enough to ignite any fuel that should fall on them.
>
> China Airlines Flight 120, August 20, 2007

China Airlines Flight 120, a regularly scheduled flight from Taiwan, landed at Naha Airport, Okinawa, Japan, at 10:26:52. The aircraft was a Boeing 737NG, with 157 passengers and 8 crew, and only five years old.

As it taxied to the stand, where three buses waited to ferry passengers to the terminal, the pilots retracted the flaps and slats that had been extended during the landing.

The driver of the bus parked farthest out on the apron watched as the 737 reached the midpoint, about fifty meters short of the end, of the line leading to the spot where the 737 would finally stop. To his surprise, he saw fuel in the form of a mist mixed in with the exhaust outflow (blast) of the engine on his side.

When the aircraft came to a stop at the set spot, the fuel continued to spray backwards as a mist, but when the engines were powered down, instead of flying backward as a mist, the leaking fuel began flowing in a stream down along the engine cowling.

Ground staff waiting at the stand noticed a liquid coming off the front of the wing, with one even catching some of it in his hand to see whether it was fuel or hydraulic fluid. But before they could issue a warning, it ignited.

Having completed the parking checklist, the captain was waiting for the ground crew member's instructions when he heard him shouting, "Fire!" Looking out of his side window, he saw thick, black smoke at the far left and behind. Even though the instruments showed no indication of fire, he actioned the extinguisher for the number one engine, and then the one for the number two engine on the right. He also ordered the cabin crew to go to their stations and prepare for evacuation. After running through the procedures, he ordered an evacuation, using Chinese, as most of the passengers were of that nationality.

The fire was burning under, and on, both wings, making use of the over-wing escape hatches out of the question, but luckily, the wind, though recorded as nine knots, was perhaps less adjacent to the terminal and at an angle of ninety degrees, blowing the flames and smoke across and not onto either the rear or front exits.

The last flight attendant to evacuate after all the passengers had was bowled to the ground just after reaching the bottom of the slide by an explosion as the fuel inside the tanks caught fire. The pilots in the cockpit had to evacuate by climbing out of the cockpit window and down an escape rope.

The first officer, who was first, was halfway down when he was blown off by the blast from the explosion. The captain followed him. Everyone had escaped, with only four people suffering relatively minor injuries. A fellow passenger had helped a woman on crutches. The cabin crew had performed well, though not many understood the instructions.

Videos (see YouTube and so on) taken from the terminal show the conflagration in its entirety, except for the moment the fire started, and demonstrate the importance of evacuating a burning aircraft as quickly as possible and not dawdling at the feet of the slides—in theory, people come down quickly, and when they slow at the bottom they end up standing up and able to run away. Everyone was evacuated from the cabins in 1.42 seconds, with both pilots out as well 14 seconds later.

The fire services only went into action six minutes after the fire was first reported to the control tower, by which time it had gained a real hold, with the back of the aircraft broken. A fearsome sight. The delay was partly due to communication failures and the distance of the fire station from the stand. Also, drivers of the appliances had to be wary of crossing areas where aircraft were operating.

Aircraft Destroyed for Lack of a Washer

The sophisticated digital flight recorder showed no electrical anomalies, there was no evidence an overheated tire was the source, and the fuel lines showed no signs of having ruptured. Therefore, the fuel the ground handler had seen coming from the right wing had to have come from the tank.

A borescope with a camera inserted into the tank soon revealed the cause of the fuel leak was a hole made by a loose bolt. It had been pushed into the thin but strong wall of the fuel tank as the powerful hydraulics retracted the slats—the bolt could be seen still lodged in the hole!

Investigators found that during a maintenance task carried out ten days before to make the slat end stop mechanism safer by putting glue on the bolt threads, a large-diameter washer—subsequently found inside the wing—had been omitted. Because of the narrow diameter of the head, there was nothing to hold it in place, and the jolt when the aircraft landed made it jump out into the confined space.

Twenty-one 737s in the US alone were found to have the same problem. The system was eventually redesigned by Boeing to prevent a reoccurrence, and existing mechanisms were replaced worldwide.

Index

Acknowledgments

Many official reports, excellent articles, and books, not to mention films of varying accuracy, have contributed to this book's realization. Twenty thousand or more items available on the Internet provided background information, at a time when it was not so easily found as now. In addition, I am sometimes citing from memory a detail or point made in now-irretrievable coverage in the local media in the countries where the incidents occurred and where I happened to be at the time.

Though it may seem ghoulish, reviewing cockpit voice recorder (CVR) transcriptions included in official reports often seemed to give a real feel to what was happening in the cockpit and a good idea of the cascading dilemmas facing the pilots.

I wasted much time, without coming to definitive conclusions, in some cases where official reports were contested as conspiratorial, as can happen when all parties—airline, manufacturer, and investigating authority, and even victims—are from the same country. Once someone claims officials have tampered with evidence, have shredded it, and are lying to boot, there is no definitive answer. From a safety point of view, this may not matter overly, as the conspirators, if any, know the truth, and stealthily, but eventually, take remedial measures.

In preparing the material, I was fortunate to come across *Air Disaster*, by the late Macarthur Job, which reviews in several volumes the most notable jet-age airliner disasters up to 1994. Job succeeds in putting them in perspective, using a wealth of technical and human detail. Those captivating volumes would be a good starting point for anyone wishing to read about a number of the pre-1995 accidents in much more detail than is possible here. Although now out of print, those books recently became available on the Kindle.

Similarly, *Disasters in the Air: The Truth about Mysterious Air Disasters*, by Jan Bartelski, was of great value in making me look again at the assumptions that had generally been made regarding some notorious disasters, and notably the worst-ever multi-aircraft disaster, in which two 747 jumbos collided on the ground in fog at Tenerife in 1977.

Some of the episodes of the excellent TV series *Air Crash Investigation*, called *Mayday* in some countries and broadcast on the National Geographic Channel among others, yielded useful new insights. Besides bringing events to life much as we have tried to do here, the highly successful series has aroused the interest of many. The producers obviously devote considerable effort, and not least money, to interviewing passengers in addition to aircrew, investigators, and experts to produce such captivating and informative videos.

At the other end of the spectrum in that it is a textbook stuffed with concentrated information regarding all aspects of aviation safety was *Commercial Aviation Safety*, by Alexander T. Wells. Its depth of detail is such that it even mentions how cockpit noise affects pilots, and in so doing helps put other safety aspects in perspective.

A Human Error Approach to Aviation Accident Analysis, by Douglas A. Wiegmann and Scott A. Shappell, was a valuable introduction to the academic work being done on accidents. Although purchased too late to be much help, I should mention *Aviation Disasters*, by David Gero, covering major civil airliner crashes since 1950. Much less discursive and opinionated than this book, it is a good tool for specialists wanting the cold bare facts concerning virtually every disaster.

Other books consulted are cited where relevant in the accounts.

While too technical for many, the Professional Pilots Network on ***http://pprune.org*** has some very interesting threads on specific topics.

The late Australian aviation journalist Ben Sandiland's *Plane Talking* blog provided leads and helpful insights on many topics, including the disappearance of MH370. Even though critically ill in hospital, he unstintingly gave advice for the second edition of this book. His outspoken and knowledgeable commentary on aviation and even astronomy will be sorely missed by many.

Investigators and other experts have proffered valuable advice and pointed out some incorrect details and given encouragement. While very appreciative, I do not mention them by name lest that give the impression they are endorsing everything said about events in which they were involved.

The official reports by air accident investigative bodies, such as the NTSB, AAIB, ATSB, BFU, and BEA, often made fascinating reading besides providing factual details.

On a personal level, I would particularly like to pay tribute to the late John Hawkins for encouraging me. His experience both as a metallurgist and as managing director and chairman of numerous companies in the British Alcan Group, developing high-temperature alloys for aircraft, including the supersonic Concorde, meant he was able to advise me about the evolution of these materials. He also informed me about some aviation incidents that although in the public domain did not make the headlines.

Others kindly read the original manuscript and gave valuable advice. They include Keith Lakin, Adrian Wojcieh, James Denny, Mike Pegler, Gerald Burke, Jonathan Evans, Hélène Bartlett, and Go Sugimoto.

Finally, I must thank Marcus Trower for copyediting this complex manuscript and Nikita Wood for kindly doing a final check.

Christopher Bartlett

Author

Christopher Bartlett initially trained as a mining engineer, a field where ensuring compliance with safety standards is of prime importance. His passion, however, has been flying, and notably air safety.

This was engendered as an air cadet during his youth and as a member of the British Interplanetary Society, as well as during sessions on fighter simulators at the Air Ministry. He completed his two years' military service in the British Royal Air Force.

After taking a degree in Modern Chinese and Japanese at the School of Oriental and African Studies, London University, he became, among other things, a professional translator of Japanese scientific and technical material. This included Japanese rocket tests. He also wrote for magazines in the Far East.

His fluency and understanding of English, French, and Japanese enabled him to undertake research based on material published in its original format and note opinions and facts that were not widely publicized. In addition, his coincidental residence in countries when and where headline air crashes occurred has enabled him to add local color and extra details to several of these accounts, and notably the worst-ever single aircraft crash, JL123, in Japan.

Table of Contents Part 2

Updates
will be placed
in
PART 3
Glossary & Flying Dictionary
(Publication September 2019)
which unlike Part 1 and 2
will have a Kindle version

How to Purchase

To find the appropriate version on Amazon go to our website ***https://chrisbart.com*** and click on the appropriated link next to the Table of Contents."

Also available from bookshops but usually must be specially ordered.

Online Shop for Multiple Copies

Flying schools, associations, clubs, and individuals wishing to buy a several copies for training or as presents, may find it very advantageous to purchase from the shop on our website ***https://chrisbart.com***. Unfortunately, we can only arrange for deliveries in the countries where the books are printed, namely Australia, the UK, and the US (Mainland).

www.ingramcontent.com/pod-product-compliance
Lightning Source LLC
Chambersburg PA
CBHW030910090426
42737CB00007B/152